Super Senses!

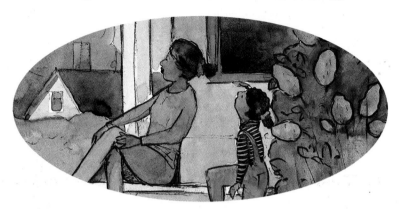

Ron Benson

Lynn Bryan

Kim Newlove

Charolette Player

Liz Stenson

CONSULTANTS

Kathyrn D'Angelo

Susan Elliott-Johns

Diane Lomond

Ken MacInnis

Elizabeth Parchment

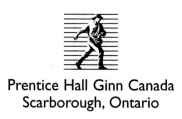

Prentice Hall Ginn Canada
Scarborough, Ontario

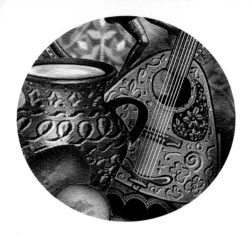

Contents

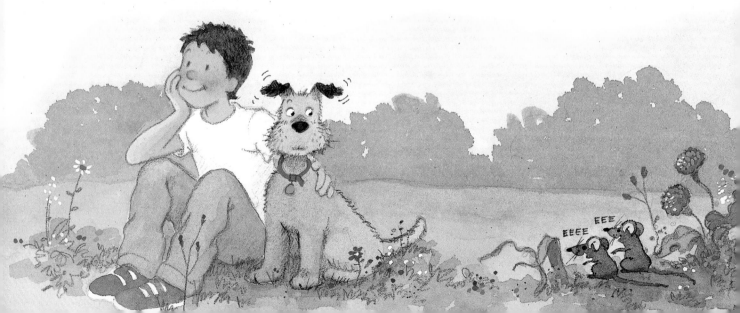

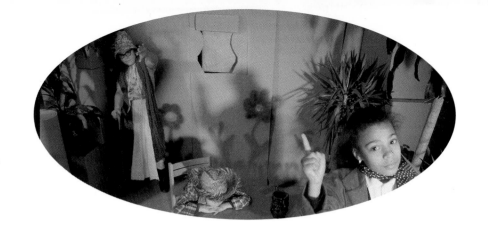

Bibliography

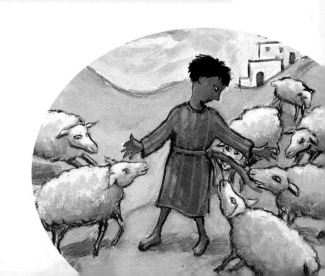

   Selections with this symbol are available on audio.

   This symbol indicates student writing.

   Canadian selections are marked with this symbol.

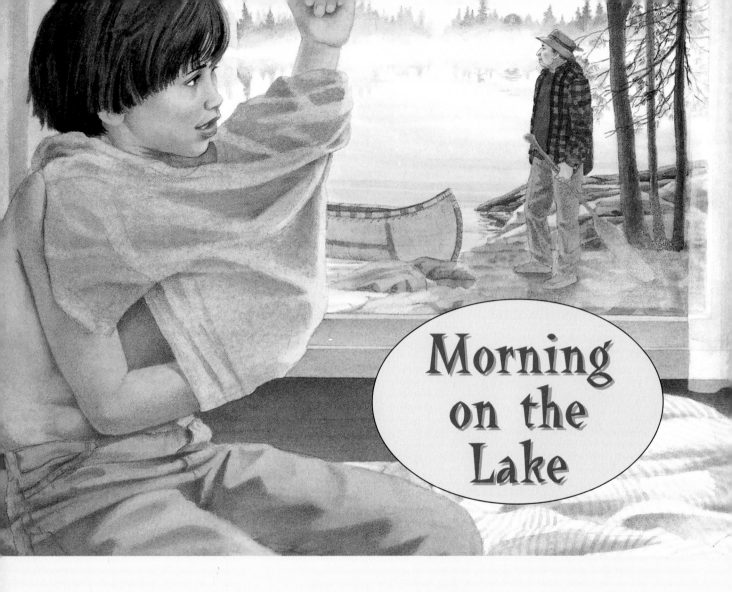

Morning on the Lake

by Jan Bourdeau Waboose
Illustrated by Karen Reczuch

"**M**orning is calling. It is time."

I hear my grandfather's slow, quiet voice in the distance. There is no need for him to say it again. I jump out of bed, rub the sleep from my eyes, and pull on my T-shirt and pants. As I run to the lake where he stands, waiting, I see his large silhouette against the pink morning sky. He is staring out at the cool, calm water. Morning mist looks like a grey blanket covering the lake. The sun is a big orange ball hiding behind the trees. I imagine it being pulled up by spiders' strings.

"I am ready, Mishomis." I yawn between the words and cover my mouth with my hand. I must be wide awake this morning.

Grandfather turns to me and smiles. He is wearing his favorite old straw hat. It has the feather of a hawk stuck in the band. I found it for him when we were walking through the bush.

On his feet are moccasins. Plain moccasins. No beads, no fur, no quills. He made them himself from moose hide. He made me a pair too, just like his.

Grandfather looks down at my feet, so I look down. I wiggle my bare toes. Grandfather slowly shakes his head from side to side. Then he grins. I grin too.

"Come, Noshen," he says in his gentle voice. He motions to the water's edge. His birchbark canoe is waiting there for us.

Long ago when I was little, I watched Grandfather make his canoe. He told me that when I was bigger I would make one just like his. I will too.

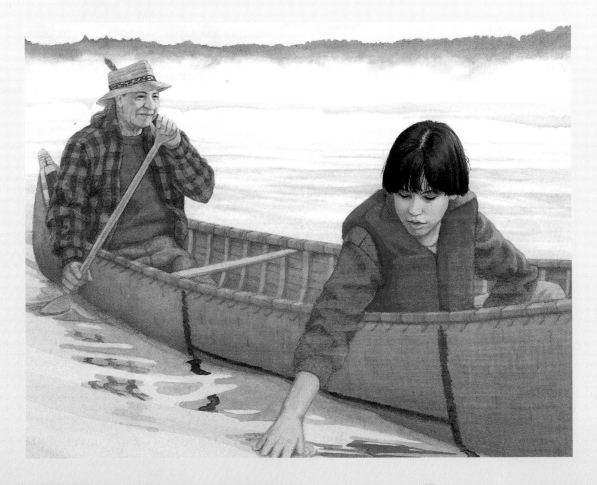

Grandfather stretches out his steady, strong arm. I hold onto it and climb into the canoe. It feels wobbly, so I sit very still. We begin to drift away from shore. Because I am in the front looking out, I cannot see my grandfather's face. But I know that he is smiling. I hear the dip of his paddle on the water and imagine many tiny bubbles trailing behind us on the glassy surface. I watch my reflection on the water as we glide.

It is still in the early morning. There is no wind and it feels cool and damp. Everything is silent, except for the sound of the paddle.

Grandfather stops the canoe in the centre of the lake. He does not speak. This is his special place. Morning is his favorite time, and so it is mine.

We wait. We listen. We peer into the thin vapors lifting from the lake. It is so very quiet that I am afraid to breathe, for I do not want to disturb this tranquil wilderness that encircles us.

Then we hear it.

A low, mellow, haunting hoot echoing across the water. And then another call and another. I shiver, but I am not cold.

"Mishomis, did you hear that?" I try to whisper but I am not quiet enough. I see

Grandfather raise his finger to his lips and then point. And I know that I must not speak again. But I cannot hold back my gasp.

There in front of us are four loons! A father and a mother with two fluffy grey babies on her back. The male loon moves closer to the canoe. He is not afraid. I wonder if I should be.

I can see the loon's white striped necklace. His shiny black back is decorated with white squares and dots.

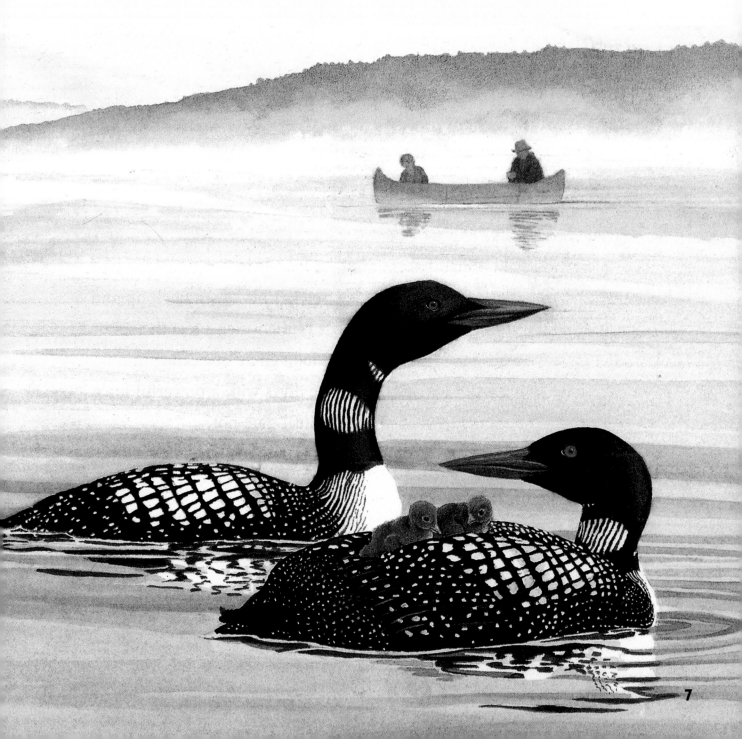

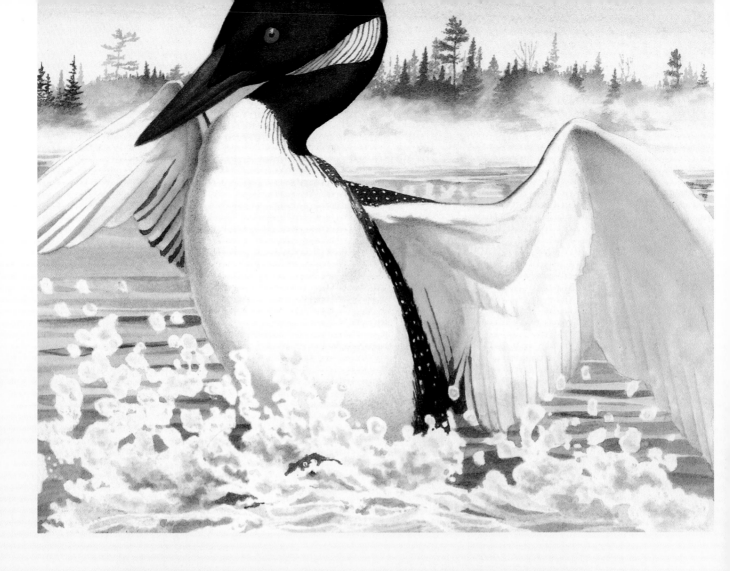

The loon is looking straight at Grandfather with his small red eyes. He stretches his silken neck up and then strikes his strong wings on the surface of the water. I feel the spray wet my shirt. I do not move as I watch the loon circle our canoe in a dance. Then, giving a sudden wild yodel, he dives with a powerful force.

My heart is pounding. I want to speak. But I dare not.

I know the loon has reminded us that the northern lake is his home. Grandfather has told me that our ancestors have given our people many stories of the Great Loon. This morning on the lake is our story.

I squint to catch a last glimpse of the family, but they have vanished. Gone, as quickly as they appeared.

The morning is no longer serene and still. Birds chirp their morning songs across the lake. I sense the animals stirring on the shore. The mist is gone. The sun, full and warm, shines bright above the trees. The wind ripples the water. The leaves sway gently in the scented breeze.

I feel that it would be all right to speak now, but I have silence on my tongue. No sound comes from the back of the canoe. I turn around to see Grandfather. He is smiling. I glance at my own reflection on the water. And I am smiling too. Just like Grandfather.

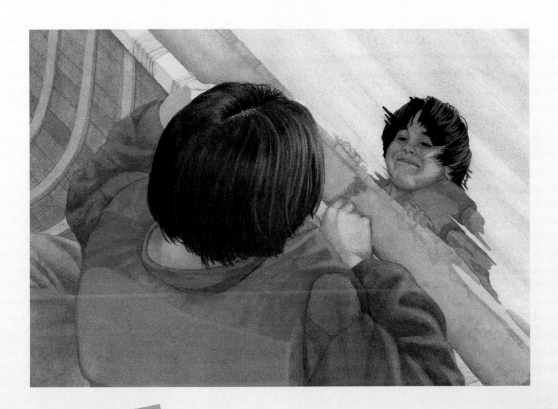

ABOUT THE AUTHOR

JAN BOURDEAU WABOOSE

Jan Bourdeau Waboose, a Nishinawbe Ojibway, grew up in northern Ontario, both on and off the reserve. She has been writing since she was seven years old. Her writing includes articles for many Native magazines and newspapers as well as poetry and short stories. She says, "What I would like people to see is that Indian people are proud, family-oriented people, respectful of all. . . ." Jan now lives in southern Ontario.

Concrete Poems

by Robert Froman

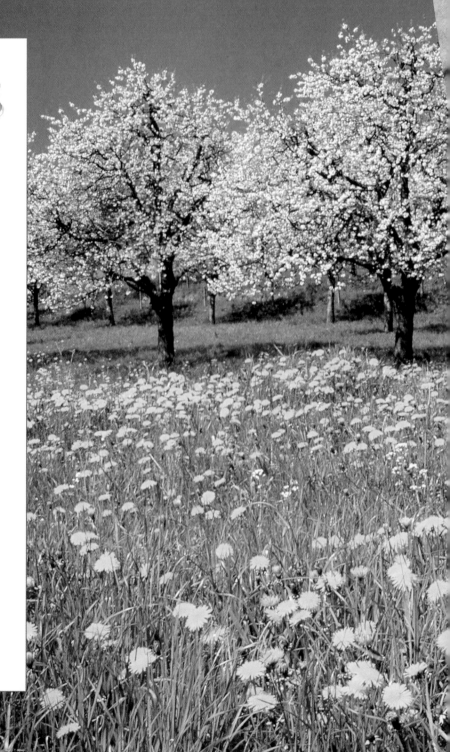

No Pretending

DANDELION, NO
BRIGHT DANDELION

You

are

not

for

any-

thing,

You

just

are.

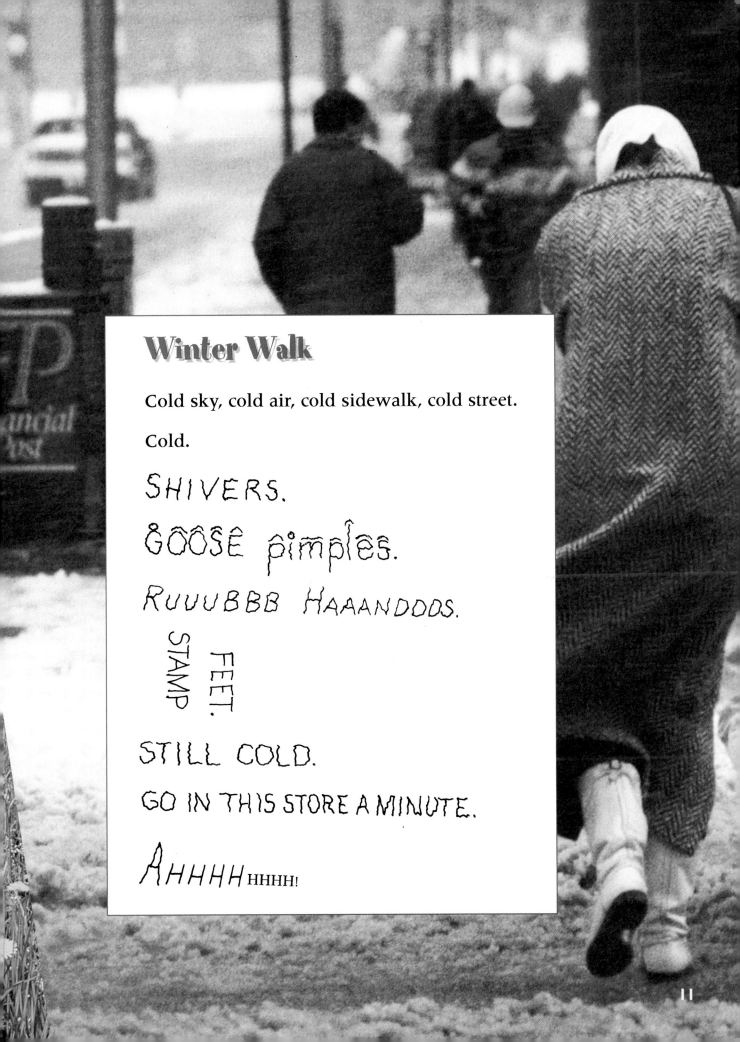

Winter Walk

Cold sky, cold air, cold sidewalk, cold street.

Cold.

SHIVERS.

GOOSE pimples.

RuuuBBB HAAANDDDS.

STAMP FEET.

STILL COLD.

GO IN THIS STORE A MINUTE.

AHHHHHHHH!

Seeing Through the Camera's Eye

Written and photographed by
Valerie Burton

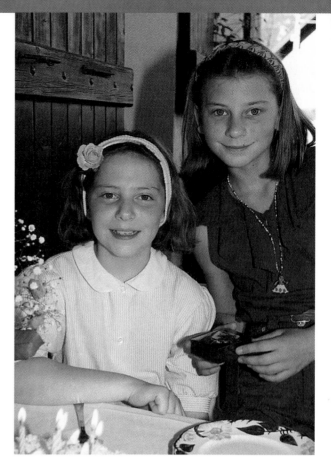

There are many reasons to take a photograph: to preserve a happy moment or to remember a special event, to have photos of friends and family, to create a beautiful picture.

People Plus

What makes a good photograph? Look at everything around you—people, animals, flowers, buildings, cars. Take time to notice all the possibilities for good pictures. You'll find interesting shapes, mysterious shadows, bright colors, and unusual patterns.

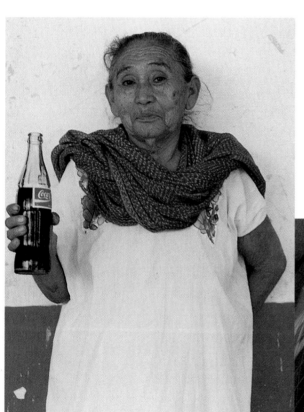

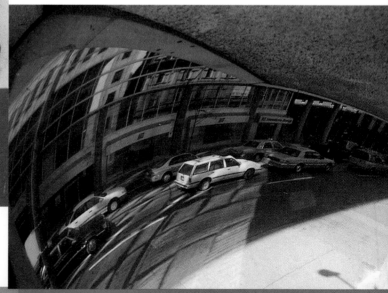

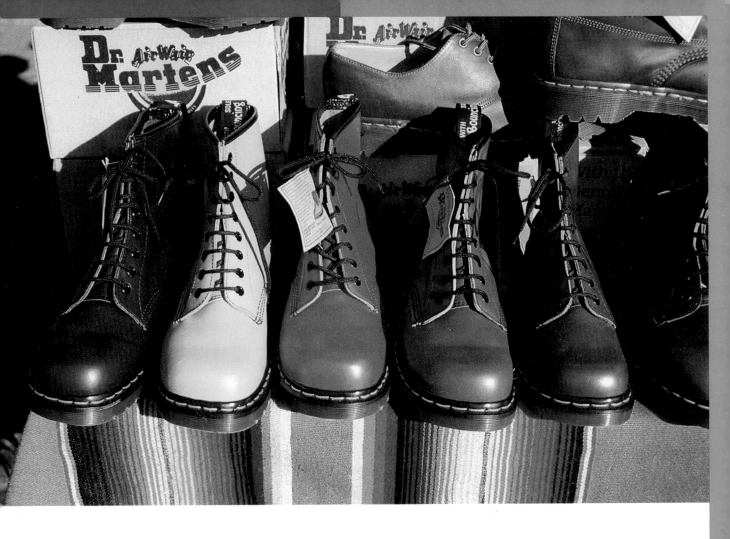

Every face is unique. Take a photograph that shows something special about someone you know well.

Walk around your neighborhood and take pictures of your favorite places and things. Try to keep your photographs as simple as possible. Concentrate on something you like, and don't put anything else in the picture.

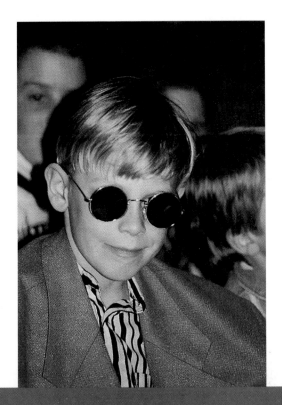

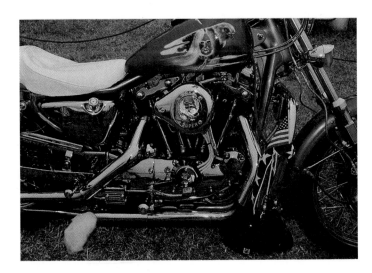

Look carefully at what you want to photograph and decide what you like most about it. If your subject is a person, it might be the eyes or the hair or perhaps the shape of the hands. A portrait doesn't have to be of a person's face.

Repeating patterns of reflections on the shiny windows can make an interesting picture.

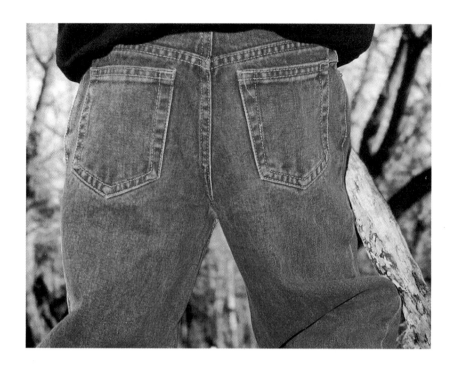

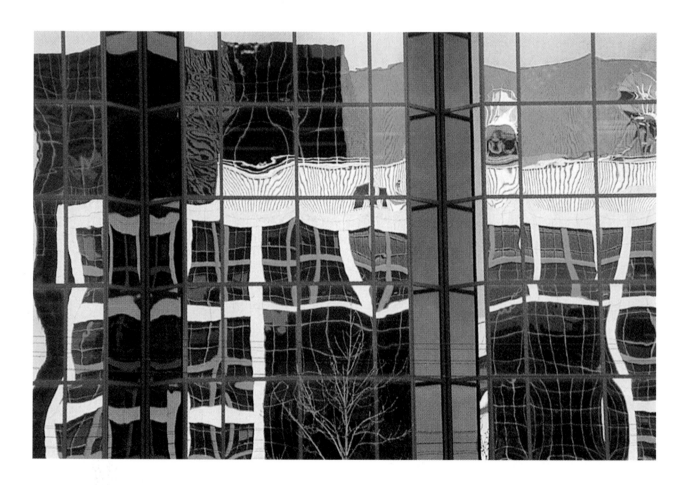

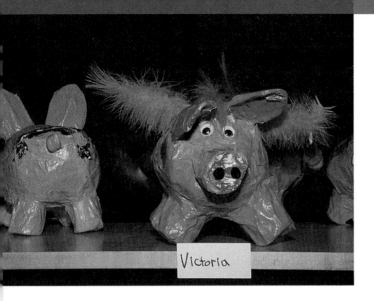

Victoria

Favorite Things

Do you like stuffed animals? What sports equipment do you use? Do you have a collection of baseball cards, stamps, comic books? What's your favorite outfit? Do you play a musical instrument? Do you have a new bike? Photographing objects can tell a story if you use your imagination.

If you create a photo album of your favorite things, you'll be able to remember them clearly in the future.

You could make a portrait of someone by taking pictures of the things they like to collect.

Take a good photograph of the person and surround the photo with a collage of pictures of their favorite things. Keep the pictures simple. Don't put too many things in the same photo. Experiment a bit with different arrangements of shapes before you take your picture. You have to choose which objects to include, what the background will be, and what camera angle to use. Start with a single, usually larger, object and then add others to complete your arrangement.

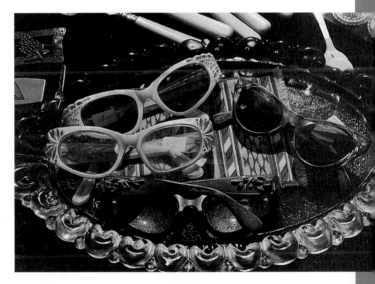

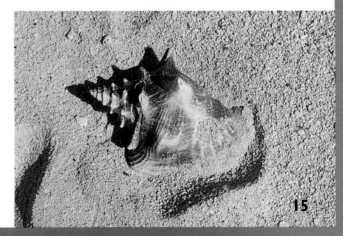

Pets and Other Animals

Try taking pictures of a day in the life of your pet. What does he or she do all day? Try to capture your pet's unique character in a photograph. Make a portrait of him or her in the same way you would photograph a friend. Use the self-timer and take a picture of the two of you together.

Some people have unusual or exotic pets in their homes. Take a picture of an unusual pet, alone or with its owner.

The zoo is a good place to take exciting pictures. Try to keep the cage bars out of your photograph.

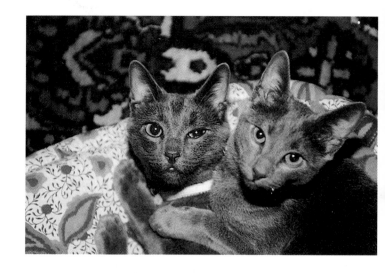

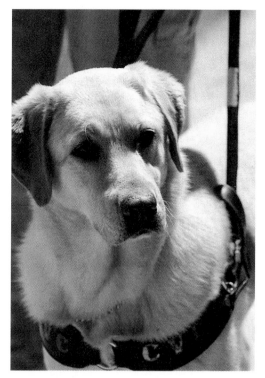

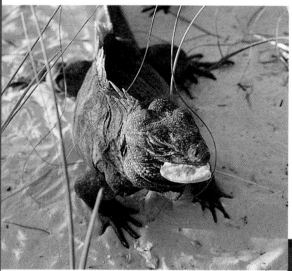

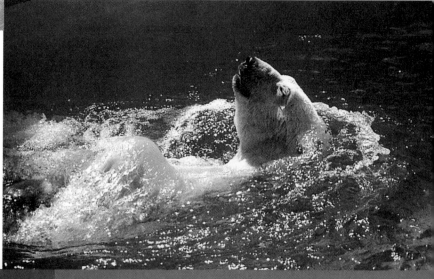

The Case of...
the Missing Skateboard

by Jeanne Iacono Martin
Illustrated by Anne Villeneuve

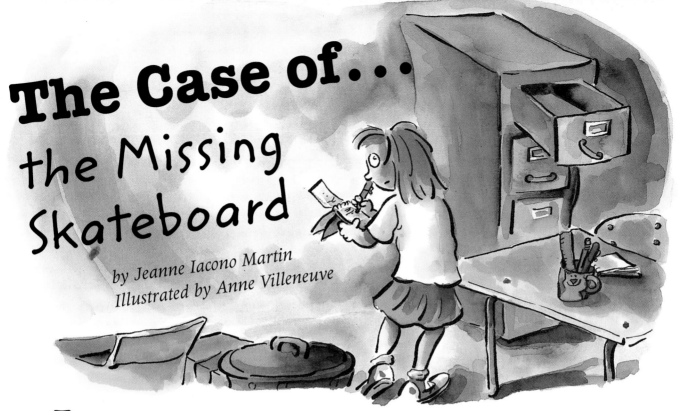

It was on the first day of summer vacation that Tracy Fletcher opened her own detective agency.

In one corner of the family garage Tracy had arranged a card table and two chairs. On the table were a notebook and several pens. Next to the table was an old file cabinet. It was empty but Tracy believed it gave her office a businesslike feeling.

Outside the garage Tracy hung her sign:

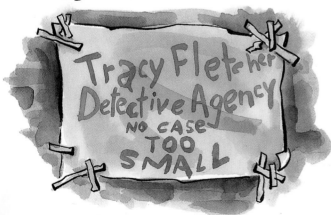

Tracy Fletcher
Detective Agency
NO CASE
TOO
SMALL

Around noon Angie Tom came into the garage. She was the best skateboarder on the block.

"He took it," Angie said, and she flopped into a chair.

Tracy grabbed her notebook and a pen. "Took what?" she asked.

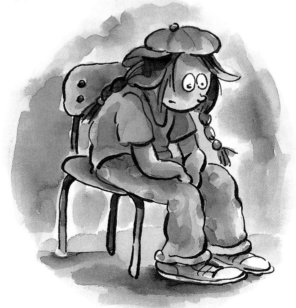

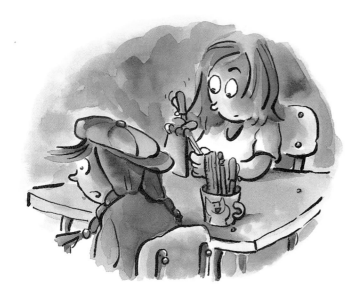

"My skateboard, of course," said Angie.

Tracy opened her notebook and wrote *Stolen—Angie's Skateboard*. "Describe your skateboard," she said.

"You've seen it!"

"I know," said Tracy, "but a complete description of a stolen object is important to a detective."

"Well, it's brown and has black grip tape," said Angie. "And David Stellino took it."

"What makes you suspect David?" asked Tracy.

"Because there is a contest at Skateboard World tomorrow. If I don't show, David will win for sure."

"Did you see David take it?"

"No, but he must have."

Tracy wrote *Suspect—David Stellino*. "I'll get right on it," she said.

"I hope you get my skateboard back before the contest," said Angie. "The winner gets a new ten-speed bike, and I sure want it."

Tracy went first to the Stellino house to question David. Mrs. Stellino answered the door.

"Hello," said Tracy. "I want to ask David if he will be entering the skateboard contest tomorrow."

"I'm afraid not," said Mrs. Stellino. "David has the chicken pox. He's been home sick for two days."

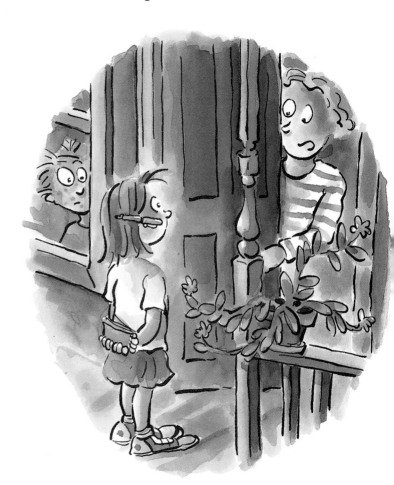

"I'm sorry to hear that," Tracy said.

Tracy walked straight down the street to Angie's house. Before she knocked, she wrote in her notebook *Suspect home with chicken pox.*

Angie and her German shepherd, Prince, came to the door. "Where's my skateboard?" asked Angie.

"Wooof!" said Prince.

Tracy patted Prince on the head. "David didn't take it. He's home with the chicken pox. This is a real mystery. Where did you last put your skateboard? There should be some clues at the scene of the crime."

Angie led Tracy to her bedroom. "There—in the corner," she said.

Tracy was a good detective. Soon she announced: "Clue number one. Here's a long brown scratch that runs down the wall."

Angie looked. "I'm sure I didn't do that."

"Probably the thief," said Tracy. "It looks as though someone grabbed the bottom end of the skateboard and it slipped right down, scratching the wall. Did you hear any strange noises?"

"Nothing."

Tracy wrote in her notebook *Clue #1—Long brown scratch.*

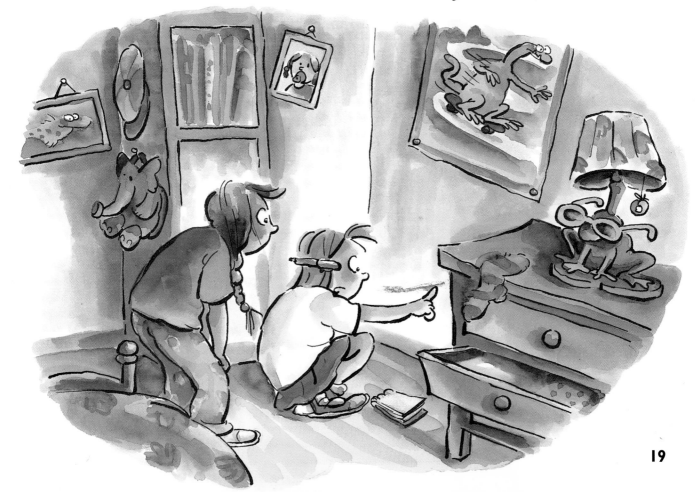

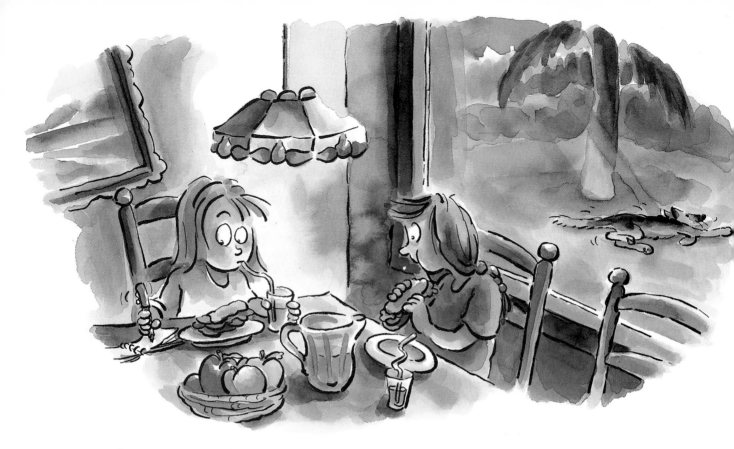

Then Tracy picked something up from the floor and handed it to Angie.

"Grass," said Angie. "It could have come from anyone's shoes. Doesn't prove a thing."

"Don't get discouraged," said Tracy. "You have a really good detective working on your case." She wrote *Clue #2—Grass.*

Angie smiled and said, "Stay for dinner."

During dinner Tracy questioned Angie more. "Was your skateboard in the corner after breakfast?"

"Yes," said Angie.

"What did you do after breakfast?"

"I wrote a letter at my desk."

"Then?"

"I took a bath. Ooooh!" squealed Angie. "It was right after my bath that I noticed my skateboard was gone."

Tracy opened her notebook and wrote *Skateboard missing after bath.* "Now we are getting somewhere," she said. "Pinpointing the time of the crime is important in solving a case."

Tracy looked out the window. Prince was rolling in the grass. She had an idea. "I want to look for more clues," she said.

In Angie's bedroom Tracy knelt down and looked closely at the floor. "Nothing more," she said. But as she was getting up

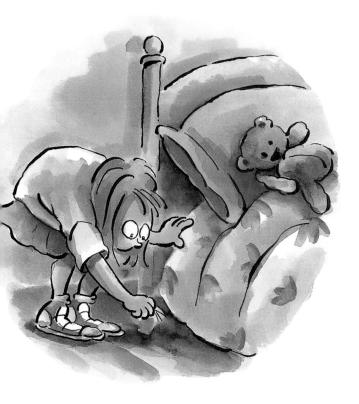

she noticed something on the bottom edge of Angie's bedspread. She picked it off. Then another. And another. She wrote *Clue #3—Dog hairs.* "I think Prince is the thief," said Tracy.

"Impossible," said Angie.

"Prince is big enough to carry a skateboard away in his mouth," said Tracy.

"Why?" said Angie.

"Jealousy," suggested Tracy. "Have you been playing with Prince enough lately?"

"Let's start looking," said Angie.

The girls searched in every room—under beds, sofas, and tables. They couldn't find the skateboard.

"You shouldn't have jumped to conclusions and accused Prince," said Angie. She went to the back door and whistled. Prince came running inside.

"I must go before it's dark," said Tracy. "Perhaps while I'm walking home I will be able to put the clues together better and come up with another lead."

Just then Prince caught sight of some birds walking across the lawn. Barking loudly, he pushed his front paws against the back screen door. The door swung open. Prince went chasing after the birds.

"That's it," said Tracy. "Prince went to your bedroom while you were bathing, picked your skateboard up in his mouth, went to the back door, pushed it open, then went outside and buried it."

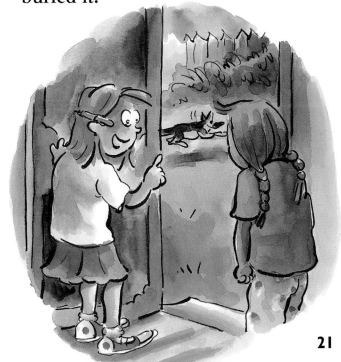

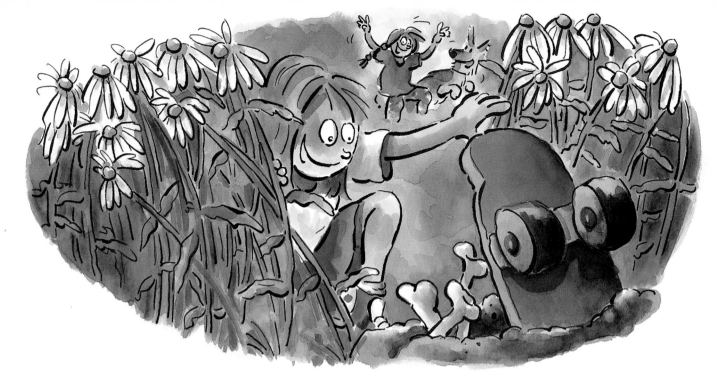

"He doesn't even bury bones. He eats them completely!"

"Let's look anyhow," said Tracy.

The girls hunted through the yard. Suddenly Tracy yelled, "Come quick, Angie."

Half-buried in a slope of daisies were dozens of old bones and one brown skateboard with black grip tape.

Angie let out a yell of delight that sounded like "Skateboard World, here I come." She picked up her skateboard.

Prince ran to her side and began barking. "OK, I'll play with you," said Angie.

"Teach Prince a new trick—like how to ride a skateboard," said Tracy.

Angie laughed. "Not a bad idea. He's a real smart dog."

Tracy opened her notebook and wrote *Case solved. P.S. Be on lookout for dog riding skateboard.*

ABOUT THE AUTHOR

JEANNE IACONO MARTIN

Jeanne Iacono Martin has taught children in both elementary and high school. She especially likes to write for children. Her work includes stories for the magazine *Highlights for Children*, the book *The Cinnamon Bear Who Wanted to Sing*, and almost a dozen coloring books. Jeanne loves going to art galleries, reading, and exploring antique shops and small country towns.

The Best Thing I Never Saw

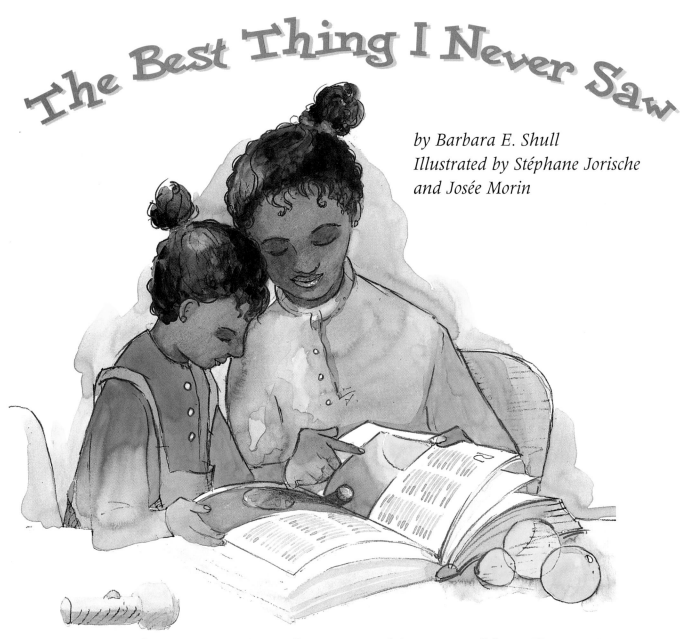

by Barbara E. Shull
Illustrated by Stéphane Jorische
and Josée Morin

Kikora was curious about everything around her. She
wanted to know the name of every tree. She learned
about the stars at night with her father. And whenever
she made a remarkable discovery, like the time she found four
white kittens in the shed, she danced with excitement.

When her mother said a total solar eclipse was coming, Kikora
wanted to learn all about it.

"A solar eclipse happens when the moon passes between the
sun and Earth. Then the moon makes a shadow on the Earth, and
it gets dark in the middle of the day," her mother explained.

"Does the shadow go away?" Kikora's eyes grew big and round.

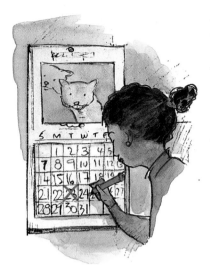

"The darkness lasts only a few minutes. Then the moon moves away from the sun. A total solar eclipse won't happen here again for a very long time," Mother said. "Next Tuesday is the big day."

Kikora was so excited, she put a big red X on the calendar. She counted the days until next Tuesday. After what seemed like forever, the big day finally came.

"What time will the eclipse happen?" Kikora asked at breakfast.

"The moon will cover the sun a little at a time. It takes about two hours," Mother answered. "The eclipse will begin around ten o'clock this morning. That means the sun should be completely covered by lunchtime."

Kikora ran to look out a window. "Clouds!" she shouted. "Nothing but clouds! I won't be able to see a thing."

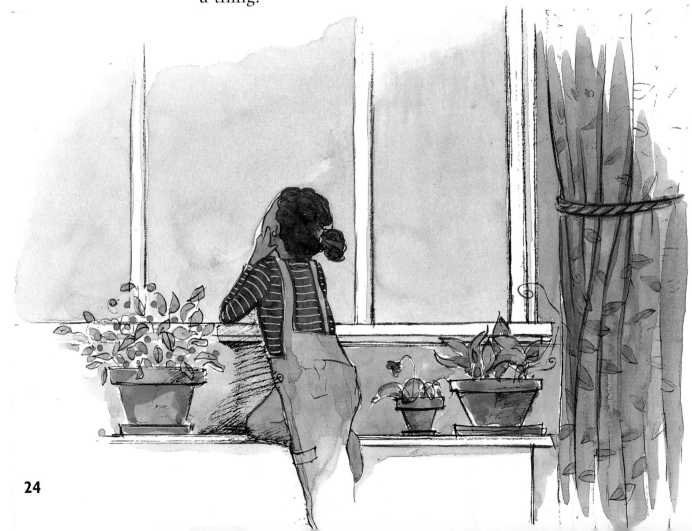

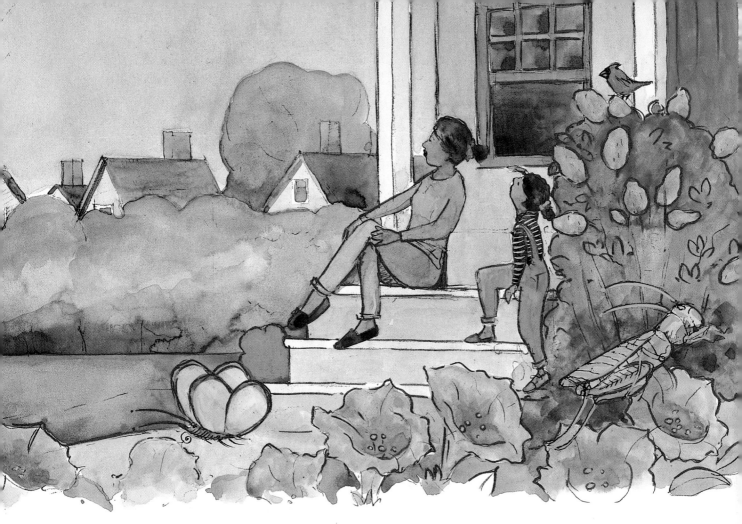

As the morning went by, the clouds stayed in the sky. Kikora wished they would drift away, but they didn't. And the longer the clouds hung overhead, the unhappier she became.

"It's twenty minutes past eleven, and nothing's happening," Kikora complained. "This is just a plain old cloudy day."

"I have an idea," Mother said. "Why don't we go out on the front porch to watch and listen for a while?"

"Watch for what?" Kikora asked.

"Just trust me and come along," said Mother.

Suddenly Kikora was curious to see what Mother meant. So she followed her mom outside and sat on the front steps. Kikora looked around at what seemed like an ordinary cloudy day. The air was damp and warm. A light breeze stirred the leaves on the trees. A yellow butterfly flitted among Mother's petunias.

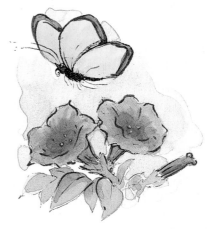

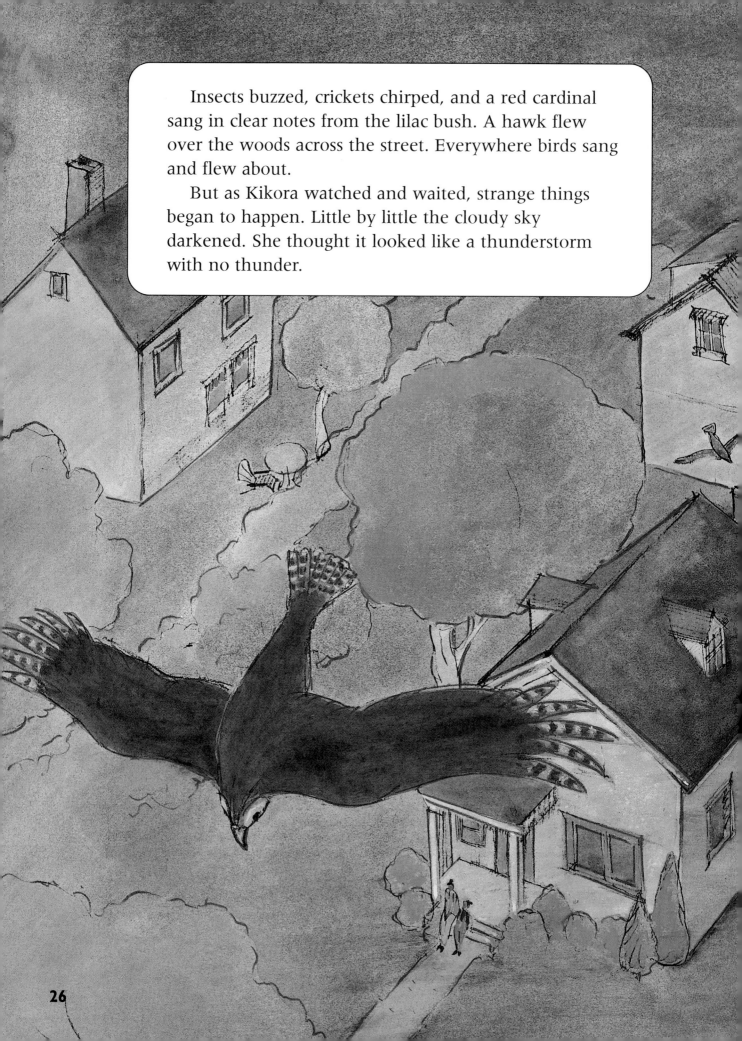

Insects buzzed, crickets chirped, and a red cardinal sang in clear notes from the lilac bush. A hawk flew over the woods across the street. Everywhere birds sang and flew about.

But as Kikora watched and waited, strange things began to happen. Little by little the cloudy sky darkened. She thought it looked like a thunderstorm with no thunder.

The cardinal in the lilac bush ended his song. All the other birds stopped singing, too. The hawk found a resting place.

As the sky grew even darker, all the insects stopped buzzing except the crickets. They chirped louder than ever. Kikora listened as an owl hooted in the woods. She shivered. She could hear her own breathing.

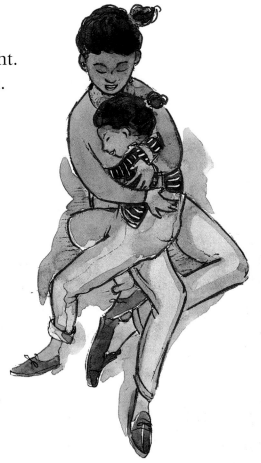

Finally, noonday became almost as dark as night. The streetlight in front of Kikora's house came on. A car went by slowly with its headlights shining. The windows in a neighboring house lit up.

But darkness lasted only a few moments. Gradually the sky lightened. Soon the cardinal began to stir. Insects resumed their activity. The chirping of crickets grew softer. As the sky grew lighter and lighter, the cardinal once again sang his song, and the yellow butterfly returned to Mother's petunias.

Kikora hugged her mother. "Did you see it? Did you see it?" she exclaimed.

"What did you see?" Mother asked.

"It's a cloudy day—I didn't really see anything. But still, it was the best thing I never saw!"

ABOUT THE AUTHOR

BARBARA E. SHULL

Barbara E. Shull was first published in the *Akron Beacon Journal* when she was ten. Later she wrote stories for magazines and newspapers, but she did not write for children until she became a grandmother. Barbara lives in Missouri with her husband and eight cats.

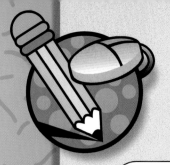

> I love writing because you can put different ideas down and get them out of your head. I think eyes are amazing things! That is why I chose to write about them.

Sight with Our Eyes

People say that sight is the most important sense after touch. You see with the pupil of your eye. The pupil is a hole in your eye. Light gets into the eye through the pupil. The pupil gets bigger if there is less light and smaller if there is more light.

Kellie Towriss
Age 9

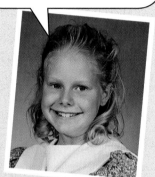

Kellie Towriss

Louis Braille's Invention

Hello! My name is Mannette. I live in a small shack in Paris. My mother is a seamstress. My father is a beltmaker. One day I was delivering one of Mother's dresses and I saw a big crowd of people around the school for boys who can't see. My neighbor, Louis Braille, went to that school so I decided to take a quick peek. I saw one of Louis' friends punching dots on a piece of paper while a teacher was reading a poem. Then Louis Braille was led out of the school and onto the platform. He skimmed his hand over the paper and read the poem to the crowd. Everyone cheered! The teacher explained how Louis had invented a system that allowed blind students to read and write. I was so proud of my neighbor, Louis Braille.

Kelsey Ireland
Age 9

> I find inventions very interesting. I also love to write!

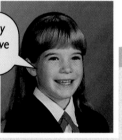

Kelsey Ireland

Speaking with Signs

by Lynn Bryan

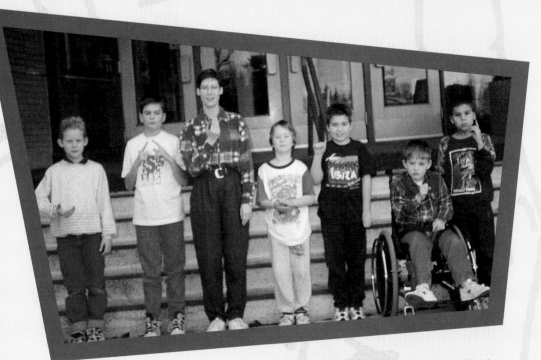

Lynn Bryan was invited to visit a Grade 3 class at the Alberta School for the Deaf. Here is what she discovered during her visit.

▲ *Theo, Mark, Autavio, Radomir, Marlow, and Errol and their teacher, Mrs. Woodard, sign a welcome.*

These six students at the **Alberta School for the Deaf (ASD)** are sending a message. They are using sign language, speaking with their hands and fingers, to say "Welcome to our school— ASD."

American Sign Language **(ASL)** is used by students and teachers at ASD, and by many people across North America.

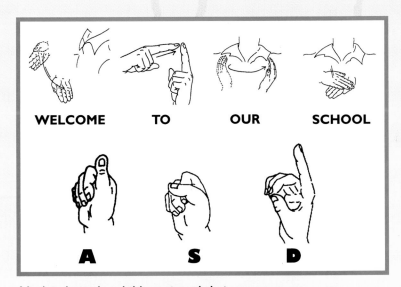

Here is how the children signed their message.

Sign Language in Action

In many ways, the classroom I visited was just like any other Grade 3 classroom. But there was one big difference. Everywhere I looked, people were speaking with signs. Signing is the children's first language—the language they use to communicate in all their lessons, conversations, and games.

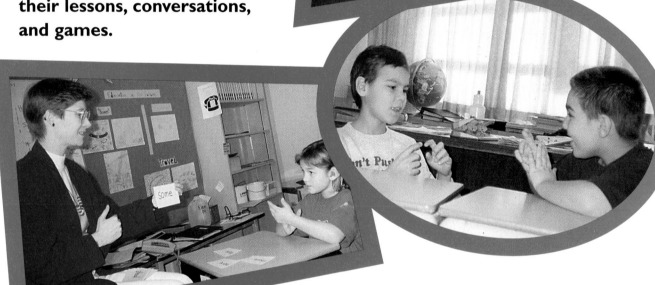

Sign language at work.

I watched their teacher, Mrs. Woodard, use sign language to explain something to Theo about his work. Then, Jessica read word cards by signing the words. Meanwhile, Marlow and Mrs. La France, the teaching assistant, used **ASL** to talk about a math question.

Errol and Radomir discussed a story they had read.

At recess time, the children signed to each other as they hurried outside to play soccer, have fun on the equipment, or just talk to their friends.

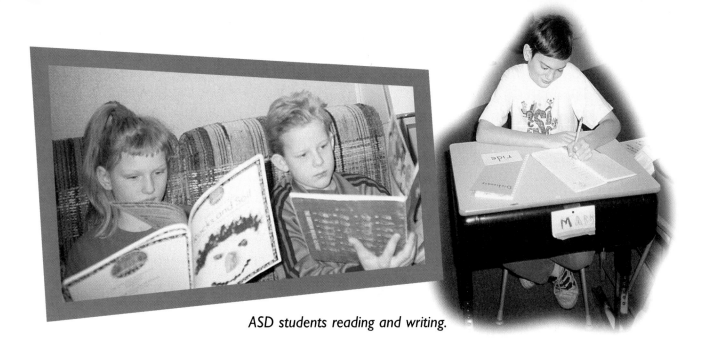
ASD students reading and writing.

Then, right after recess, the Grade 4 and 5 class invited all the elementary classes into the drama room to watch a play. They had made the play up themselves, and all the characters' words were signed.

Just before lunch, the children worked on stories they were writing or read books from their classroom library. Students at ASD learn to read and write English. Some of them also take speech classes. It must be hard work learning a language when you can't hear the words!

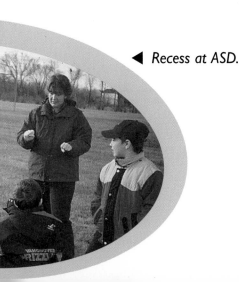

◀ Recess at ASD.

Special Inventions for Special Needs

At home and at school, ASD students use the telephone and TV set in special ways. After lunch, Autavio showed me how he uses a special phone with a keyboard. First he typed his message on the keyboard. The words went over the phone lines to the phone of the person he had called.

A student using the telephone keyboard. ▶

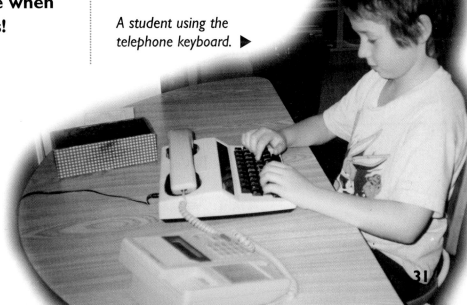

There the words would move across the phone's display screen and be printed out on paper. Just above Autavio, there was a white light on the wall. That light flashes to show that there's an incoming call.

Later in the afternoon, the children watched an educational TV program. Their TVs have a special decoder. They print the words being said at the bottom of the screen. These words are called "closed captions." Television guides mark captioned programs with "CC" or the ⬚ symbol. You can also get videos with closed captions. Some programs use a different system.

An interpreter signs the words as the program is being filmed, and the signing appears in the corner of the TV screen.

I spent a really exciting day at the Alberta School for the Deaf. When it was time for me to go, all the children were busy doing social studies. Mrs. Woodard got their attention by turning the light switch off and back on. They looked up, smiling. I smiled back, waved good-bye, and used the sign that means "thank you."

Sign for "thank you."

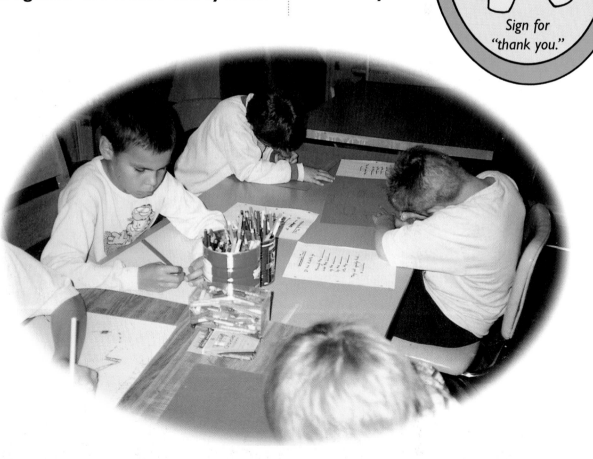

32

Too Much Noise

by Christel Kleitsch
Photographed by Gilbert Duclos

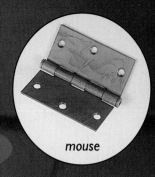
mouse

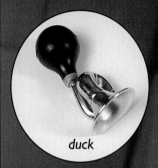
duck

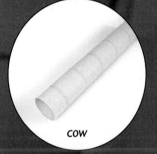
cow

Characters:

Narrator
Farmer Fred
Wise Woman

Props: noisemakers

squeaky hinge or something
   else that makes a squeaky
   sound (mouse)
bicycle horn to blow (duck)
paper towel roll to "moo"
   through (cow)
2 wooden blocks to bang
   together (horse)
2 sandpaper blocks to rub
   together (chickens)

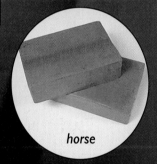
horse

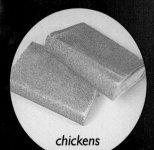
chickens

*The Narrator is standing off to the side. Farmer
Fred is lying down on his bed in his little house.*

Narrator
Once upon a time there was a farmer
named Farmer Fred who lived all alone in a
little house.

Farmer Fred lifts up his head and waves—

Farmer Fred
That's me.

Narrator

Quiet over there, Farmer Fred . . . Well, one night that farmer was tired, very tired, after working all day long on his farm. But he couldn't go to sleep.

The Narrator peeks over at Farmer Fred. He is lying still on his bed as if asleep.

Narrator *(louder)*

He just couldn't go to sleep.

Still no action from Farmer Fred. His eyes are closed.

Narrator

He was *tossing and turning* in his bed.

Farmer Fred starts tossing and turning.

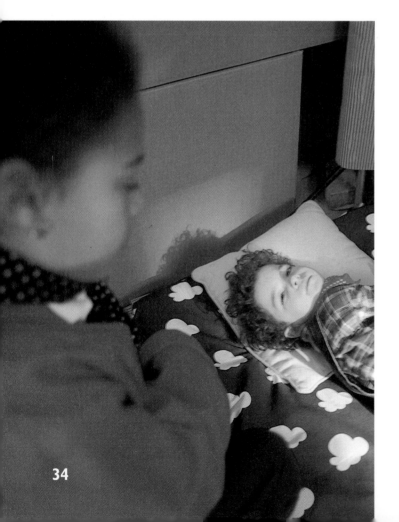

Narrator

That's better . . . And the reason the farmer couldn't sleep was because of a little mouse.

Farmer Fred moves the hinge—squeak! Then poor frustrated Farmer Fred sits up and holds his ears closed.

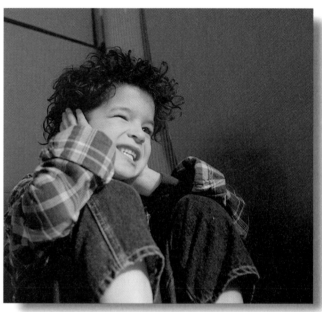

Narrator

The mouse was inside the walls of the farmer's house and that mouse squeaked all night long. So Farmer Fred decided to go to the village to see the Wise Woman.

Farmer Fred gets up and stretches. He goes to the Wise Woman.

Farmer Fred

Wise Woman, please help me! I can't go to sleep because a mouse in my house is squeaking all night long.

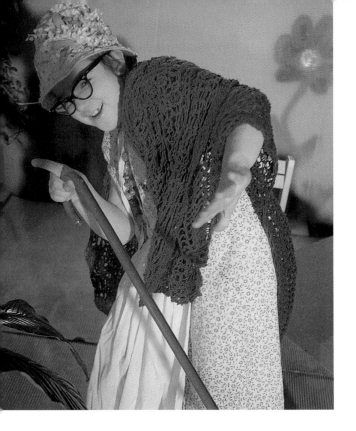

Wise Woman sings this verse rap-style.

Wise Woman *(sings)*
YOU GOT TROUBLE WITH A
MOUSE?
YOU GOT TROUBLE WITH A
MOUSE IN YOUR HOUSE?
WELLL . . .
WHEN YOU GOT TROUBLE WITH
A MOUSE IN YOUR HOUSE,
WHAT YOU NEED IS A COW—
GET A COW!
GO ON RIGHT NOW AND GET A
COW
INTO THAT HOUSE WITH THAT
MOUSE.

Farmer Fred *(amazed)*
A cow? In the house?

The Wise Woman nods. Farmer Fred shrugs.

Farmer Fred
If you say so.

Farmer Fred goes back to bed and lies down.

Narrator
So the next night before the farmer went to sleep he brought his cow into the house.

Farmer Fred blows the bicycle horn. The Wise Woman shakes her head.

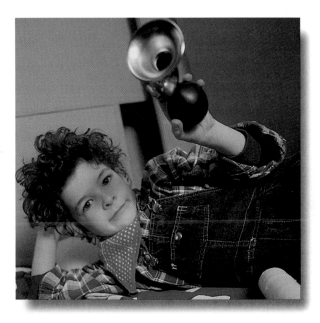

Wise Woman
The cow! The cow!

Farmer Fred gets out the paper towel roll. He puts his mouth to it and says—

Farmer Fred
MOOO.

Then Farmer Fred squeaks the hinge. He covers his ears with his hands and makes a frustrated face.

Narrator

But now the cow and the mouse were both keeping Farmer Fred awake. So back he went to the Wise Woman.

Farmer Fred goes to the Wise Woman.

Farmer Fred

Wise Woman, please help me! I brought that cow into my house like you told me. But now the cow is mooing and the mouse is squeaking and I *still* can't sleep!

Wise Woman *(sings)*

YOU GOT TROUBLE WITH A COW?
RIGHT NOW, YOU GOT TROUBLE WITH A COW?
WELLL . . .
WHEN YOU GOT TROUBLE WITH A COW RIGHT NOW,
WHAT YOU NEED IS A HORSE—
GET A HORSE!
GO ON, MY FRIEND, GET A HORSE, INTO THAT HOUSE WITH THAT COW, AND THAT MOUSE.

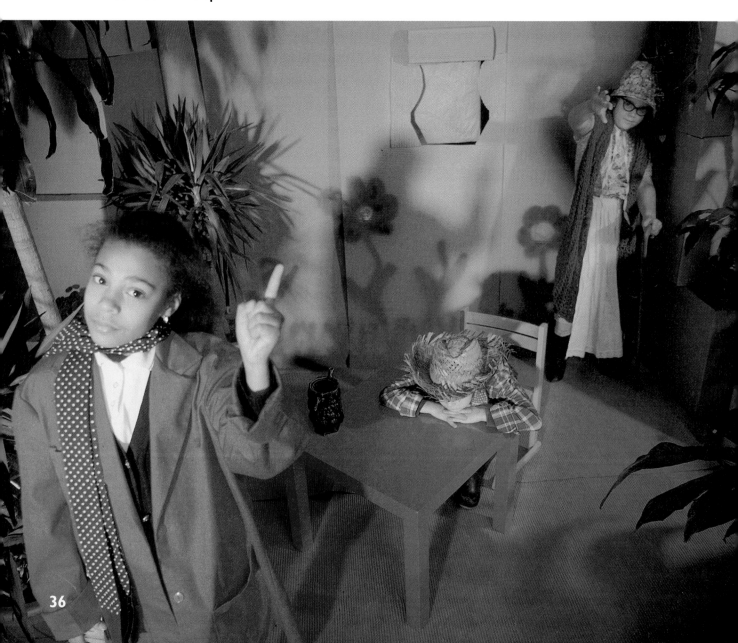

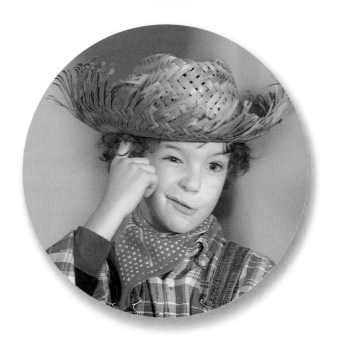

Farmer Fred
A horse?!? Well—

Farmer Fred goes back and lies down.

Narrator
The farmer did what the Wise Woman told him. And the next night the mouse squeaked, the cow mooed, *and* the horse stomped with his big hoofs—

Farmer Fred does the sound effects in the wrong order: bangs the wooden blocks together, squeaks the hinge, mooos into the paper towel roll. The Narrator gives him a long-suffering look.

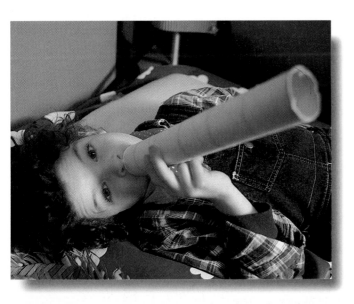

Narrator
—and the poor farmer *still* couldn't sleep. So back he went to the Wise Woman and told her his problem.

Farmer Fred gets up and goes to the Wise Woman.

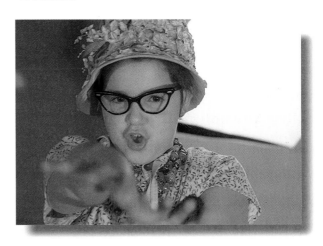

Wise Woman *(singing)*
YOU GOT TROUBLE WITH A HORSE?
YOU SAY OF COURSE, I GOT TROUBLE WITH A HORSE!
WELLL . . .
WHEN YOU GOT TROUBLE WITH A HORSE, OF COURSE
WHAT YOU NEED IS A DUCK—
GET A DUCK!
GO ON RIGHT NOW AND GET A DUCK,
INTO THAT HOUSE WITH THAT HORSE, AND THAT COW, AND THAT MOUSE.

Farmer Fred *(upset)*
A duck! A duck will quack all night long! How's that going to help?!?

Wise Woman *(sternly)*

But the farmer listened to the Wise Woman.

Farmer Fred

I don't think a duck is going to work! No way!

Wise Woman *(stronger this time)*

The farmer *listened* to the Wise Woman.

Farmer Fred trudges back to his bed and lies down.

Narrator

But the next night his house was noisier than ever.

Farmer Fred does the sound effects of all the animals: squeaky hinge, paper towel roll, wooden blocks, and bicycle horn. He keeps going for longer than the Narrator thinks he needs to.

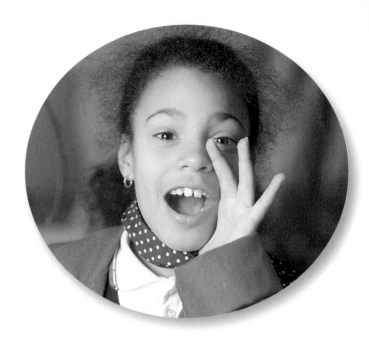

Narrator *(loudly over his racket)*

So back he went to the Wise Woman and this time she said—

Farmer Fred trudges toward the Wise Woman and before he even reaches her, she begins her advice. Farmer Fred shakes his head in despair and turns back to his home.

Wise Woman *(sings)*

YOU GOT TROUBLE WITH A DUCK?
YOU GOT NO LUCK, YOU GOT
TROUBLE WITH A DUCK?
WELLL . . .
WHEN YOU GOT NO LUCK,
TROUBLE WITH A DUCK, WHAT
YOU NEED
IS SOME CHICKENS—
GET SOME CHICKENS!
GO ON RIGHT NOW, GET SOME
CHICKENS,
INTO THAT HOUSE WITH THAT
DUCK, AND THAT HORSE, AND
THAT COW, AND THAT MOUSE.

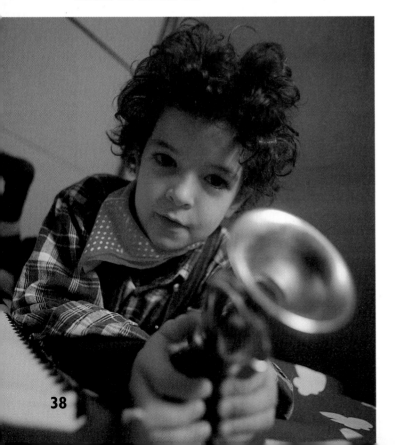

Farmer Fred goes and lies down again. He makes all the animal noises: squeaky hinge, paper towel roll, wooden blocks, bicycle horn, and rubs the sandpaper blocks together. Then he gets up and runs back to the Wise Woman again, hands over his ears.

Farmer Fred

I can't sleep! I can't sleep! How can I sleep with all those animals in my house?

Wise Woman

Well . . . I've got another idea . . . How about if you take all those animals *out* of your house?

Farmer Fred *(brightening)*

All of them? Out of the house?

The Wise Woman nods. Farmer Fred runs back home joyfully, throws away all the noisemakers except the hinge and lies down again.

Narrator

So the next night when the farmer went to bed, that little mouse—

Farmer Fred squeaks the hinge but keeps on sleeping.

Narrator

—didn't really seem noisy at all. And Farmer Fred fell fast asleep—in a minute . . . And that's the end.

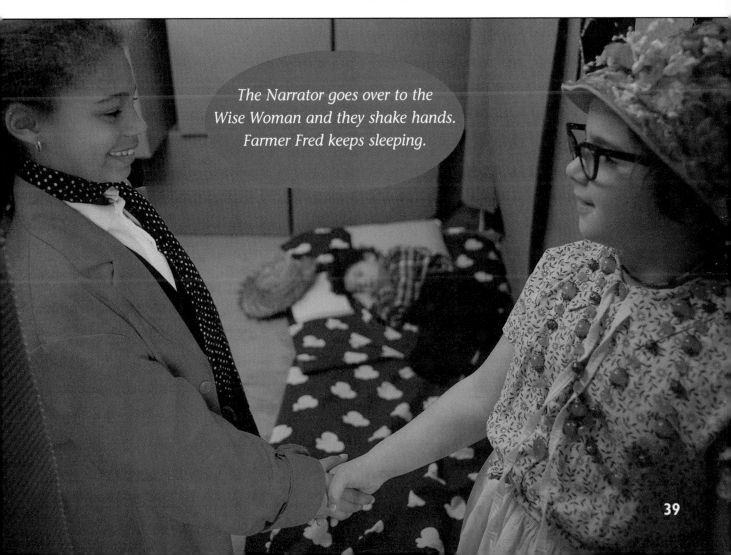

The Narrator goes over to the Wise Woman and they shake hands. Farmer Fred keeps sleeping.

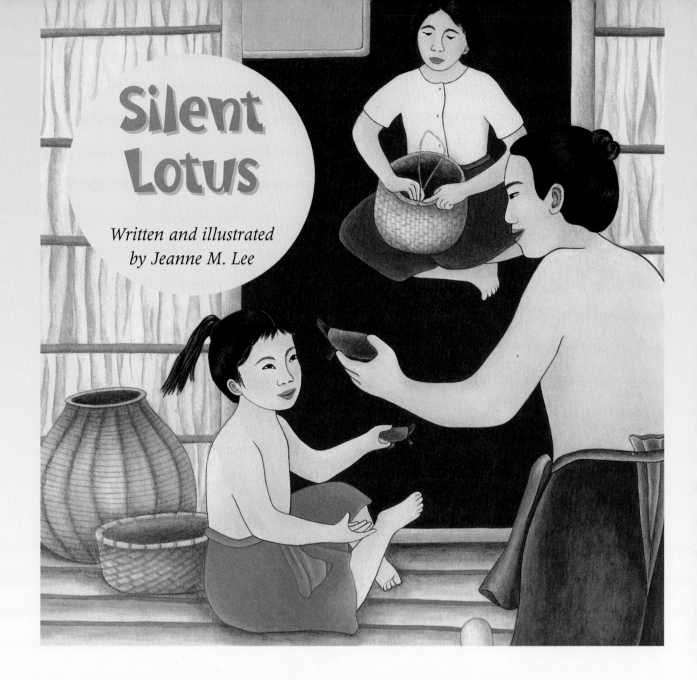

Silent Lotus

*Written and illustrated
by Jeanne M. Lee*

Long ago in Kampuchea, a man and woman lived on the edge of a lake. A daughter was born to them. She was beautiful, with a face as round as the moon and eyes as bright as the stars.

The father and mother named her Lotus, like the blossoms that covered the lake. They were very happy with their baby, for she was as good as she was lovely.

Years went by, but Lotus was as silent as on the day she was born. When she was sad tears would fall from her eyes, and when she was happy smiles would light her face.

Her father and mother knew that Lotus could not hear. She could not learn to speak. They prayed to the gods, hoping they would take this misfortune away, and cherished their daughter even more.

One day, the mother and father pointed to the blossoms on the lake and to Lotus. Then the mother put her palms together with her fingers bent, forming a flower. Lotus understood. She copied her mother's gesture and so learned to name herself with her hands.

Lotus grew lovelier each day. She liked to weave baskets out of the tall grasses that grew around the lake and to swim with the turtles while her father fished. But Lotus was happiest when she walked among the herons, cranes, and white egrets, joining them in their graceful steps.

Yet Lotus would often sit by herself, lonely and sad. She wanted so much to play with the other children. But if she motioned to them, they pretended not to see. If she pulled their arms to get their attention, they ran away.

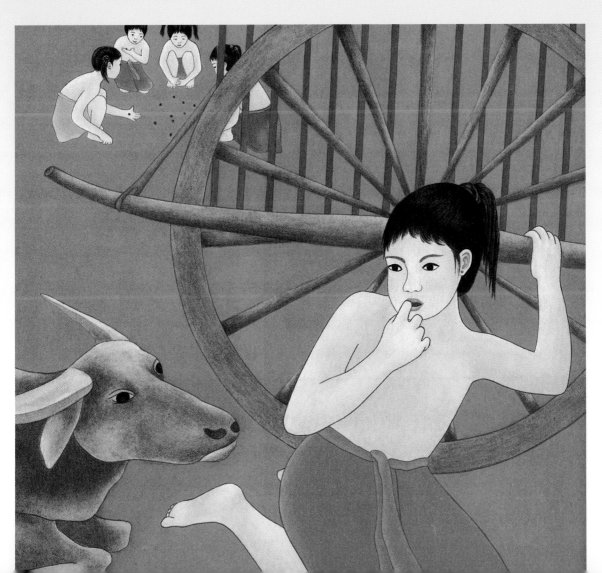

Her father and mother saw her unhappiness, but they did not know how to help her. They hoped for a sign from the gods.

Finally, they decided to go to the temple in the city. The mother put wild rice and lotus flowers in a basket as offerings; the father carried his precious daughter on his shoulders. They walked through many fields and villages, and over many canals.

When they reached the city, they hurried to the temple. Inside, the father and mother heard drums and cymbals. Lotus felt the vibrations. Then two lines of dancers appeared.

Elbows high and knees bent, Lotus imitated their movements. Long after the dancers had gone, the little girl danced. Her father and mother looked at each other. It was the sign they had hoped for.

They went to the palace. There, the queen noticed the lovely little girl and whispered to the king.

"Speak," the king said, pointing to Lotus.

"Our daughter does not speak or hear," her father said. "But she would learn to dance."

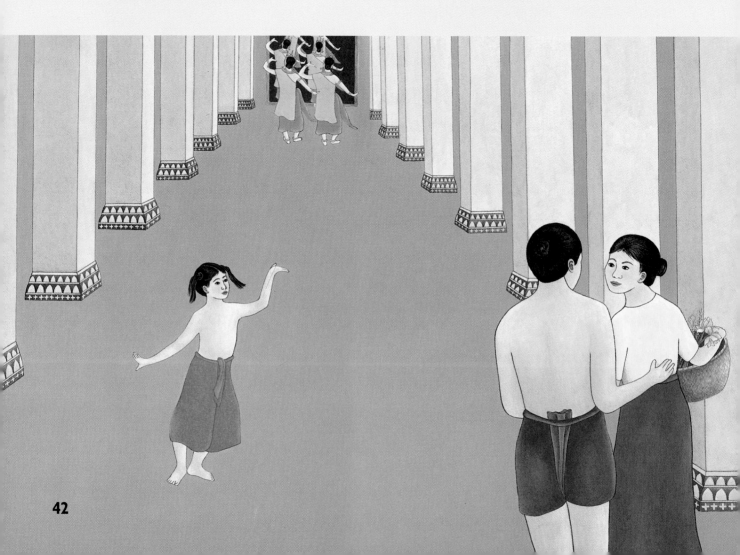

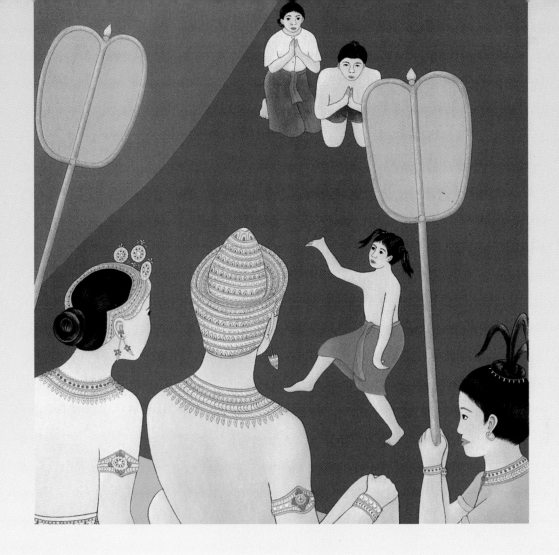

The mother motioned to her young daughter. Lotus began to dance the way she knew best, like the herons, cranes, and white egrets. The king and queen watched with delight.

"She is a most beautiful child," said the queen.

"She will learn to dance," said the king.

In the dance pavilion on the palace grounds, a graceful old woman taught Lotus how to dance the tales of the gods and kings.

Patiently, she guided the young dancer, showing her the movements that would tell those tales. Lotus learned to curl her fingers backwards and to bend her elbows and knees.

As time passed, silent Lotus began to speak with her hands, body, and feet. She loved to dance the tales of the gods and kings. And as she grew, the movements became as natural for her as the dances of the birds.

Lotus made many friends. She was no longer lonely and sad.

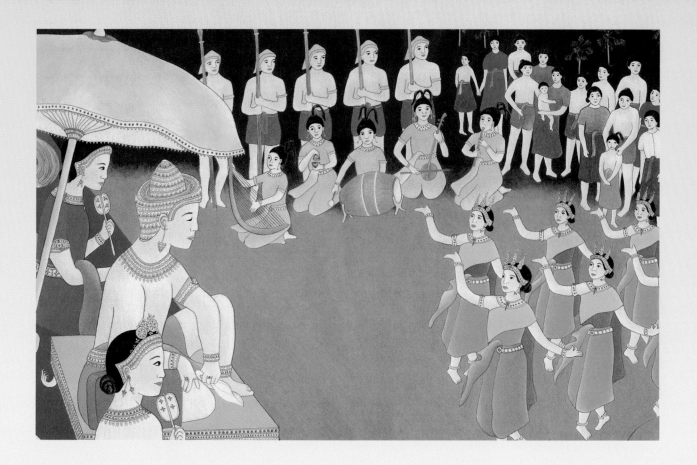

Finally, she was ready to dance for the king again. The court ladies dressed her in the brightest silks. They adorned her hair with gold and jasmine flowers. On her neck, arms, wrists, and ankles they put bands of precious stones and pearls.

It was the first night of the new year. Lotus danced better than she ever had, and as she danced, she saw pleasure and delight in the eyes of the people.

It was said that Lotus became the most famous dancer in the Khmer kingdom, dancing in the king's court and in the temples of the gods.

ABOUT THE AUTHOR JEANNE M. LEE

Jeanne M. Lee has worked as a freelance graphic artist, and her paintings have been shown in New Jersey and Boston. She has travelled in Europe and the United States. Jeanne has also visited and lived in many parts of Southeast Asia, including China.

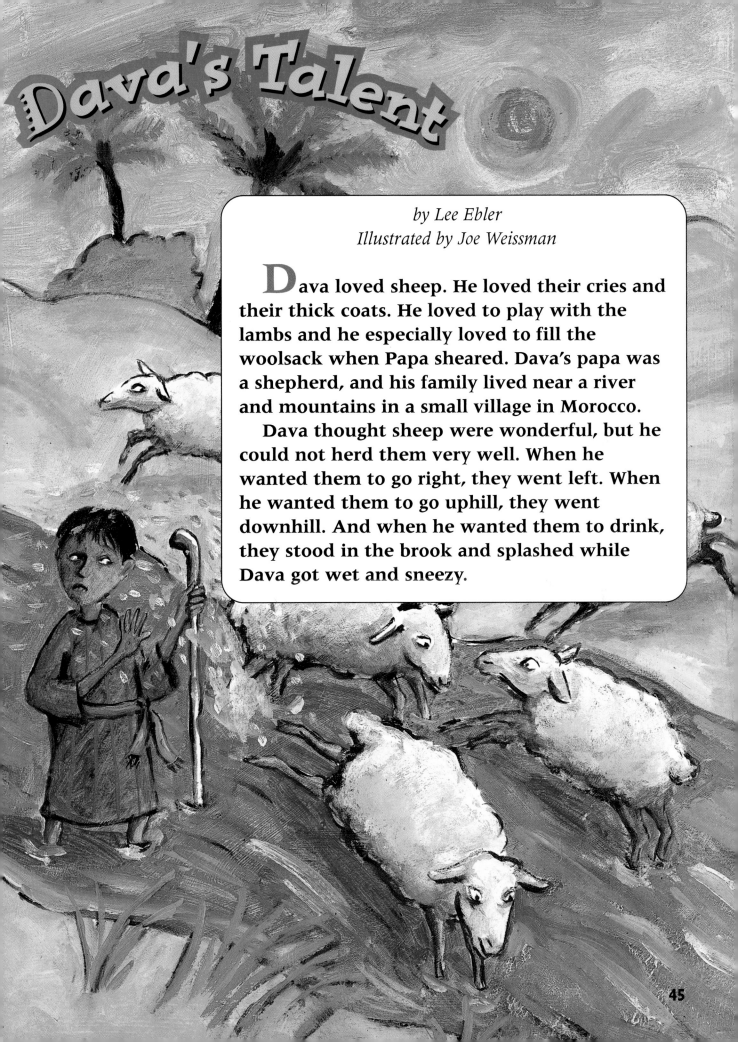

Dava's Talent

by Lee Ebler
Illustrated by Joe Weissman

Dava loved sheep. He loved their cries and their thick coats. He loved to play with the lambs and he especially loved to fill the woolsack when Papa sheared. Dava's papa was a shepherd, and his family lived near a river and mountains in a small village in Morocco.

Dava thought sheep were wonderful, but he could not herd them very well. When he wanted them to go right, they went left. When he wanted them to go uphill, they went downhill. And when he wanted them to drink, they stood in the brook and splashed while Dava got wet and sneezy.

"All your forefathers have been shepherds," said Uncle Eban. "Why won't the sheep obey you?"

"I don't know," said Dava sadly.

"Maybe if you wear Papa's clothes," suggested his sister Leah, "the sheep will think you're Papa and mind you."

So Dava put on Papa's djellabah. The sleeves covered his hands, and the hem dragged on the ground. When he walked toward the sheep, he tripped and fell. The sheep were not fooled. While Dava struggled out of the djellabah, they got into the garden and ate the melons.

"Perhaps you should walk slower when you lead the sheep," said Mama. "Sheep do not like bouncy shepherds."

So Dava walked slowly. But he was so slow that the sheep thought he was a tree. They chewed on his sash, leaving it sticky and shredded. Dava decided that walking slowly wasn't the answer.

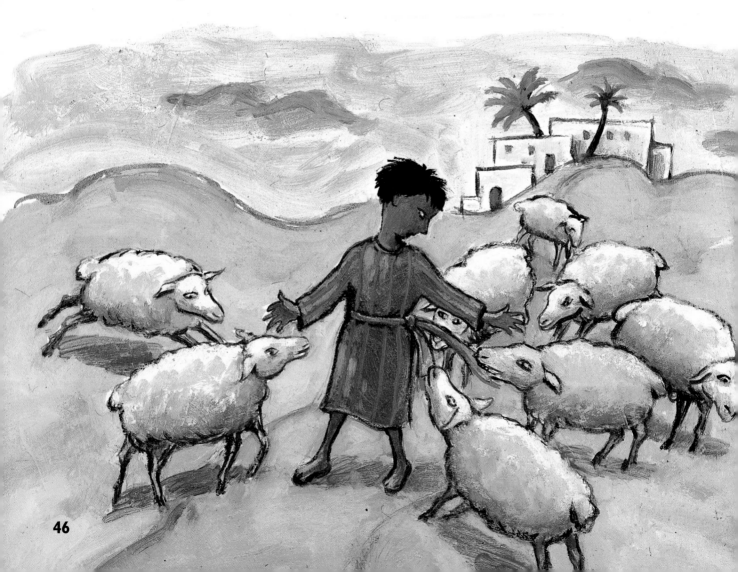

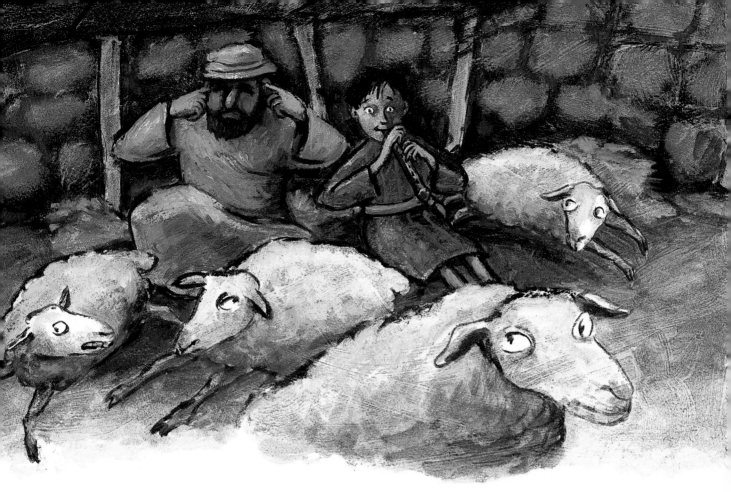

"Every shepherd has a talent to offer," said Papa.
"When you find yours, the sheep will obey. Uncle Eban
plays the flute. My talent is singing. We both lead the
herd with our music."

"Maybe I'm a singer like Papa," said Dava to Bright
Eyes, the smallest sheep. He began to sing in a loud voice
about streams and green grass. He thought he had found
his talent until Leah chased him away from the house.

"Your music sounds like rocks falling!" she said,
slamming the door.

"I will loan you my flute," said Uncle Eban. "It's clear
that you are not a singer."

So Dava played the flute. He practised inside the
sheepcote until Uncle Eban stuck wool in his ears and
the sheep began to bleat. They did not like his flute
playing.

"You screech like a hawk!" said Uncle Eban, taking
back the flute. "You're scaring the sheep."

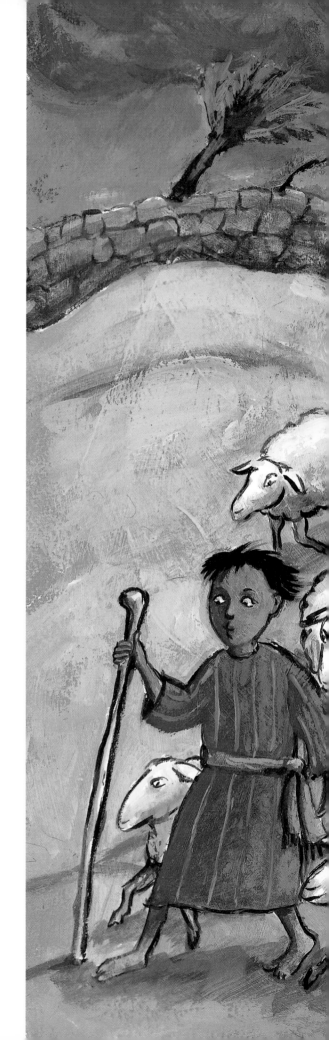

"I will never be a good shepherd," said Dava to Bright Eyes.

One day a terrible thing happened. Papa and Uncle Eban were repairing the stone wall. They were working fast because a storm was coming. Suddenly one of the rocks fell on Papa's foot. Dava could see that it hurt. He started toward Papa, but Uncle Eban stopped him.

"I'll take your papa home, but you must lead the sheep back by yourself. Take them slowly, as you have learned."

"But I can't," said Dava. "The sheep won't listen to me."

"Please try," said Uncle Eban.

Dava watched Papa and Uncle Eban leave. The sky was getting dark, and the wind was rising. The sheep began to bleat.

Dava picked up the staff and swished it around. "Hoy!" he shouted. "Hoy, Trud and Bright Eyes. Hoy, Spots!"

But the sheep did not listen. Thunder echoed over the mountains, and the frightened sheep moved toward the broken wall. If Dava didn't stop them, they would run into the desert.

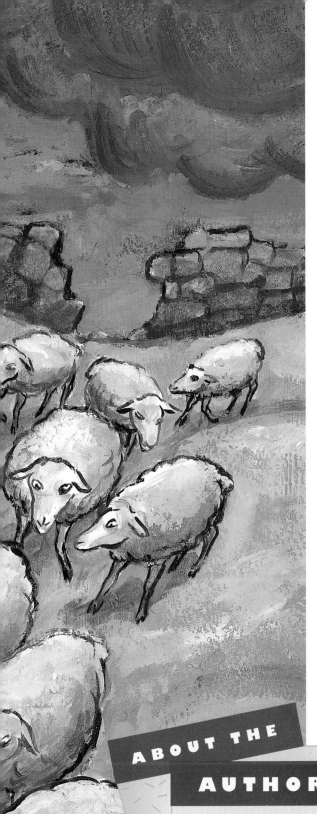

Almost without thinking, Dava began to whistle softly. The sheep didn't hear it, but the whistle calmed Dava. So he whistled louder. Beside him, Bright Eyes stopped trembling.

Then Dava had an idea. He stood in the centre of the herd and whistled. He whistled a hopeful tune, a cheerful tune, an everything's-all-right tune. And the sheep understood. They grew calm, because Dava was calm. Still whistling, Dava led them toward the sheepcote. He knew the sheep trusted him now. He felt as if he were part of the flock.

I am a whistler, thought Dava, smiling.

The sheep came safely home that day, and Papa was soon feeling well enough to hear Dava's story.

ABOUT THE AUTHOR LEE EBLER

Lee Ebler has been writing for ten years and has been published in nearly thirty magazines. She says that the idea for "Dava's Talent" came because she "loves sheep—they were one animal we didn't have while growing up on the farm. . . . I was also thinking of how individualized talents are, and yet, sometimes we have to work to discover them in ourselves."

"Sounds" Like Fun

by Barbara Shapiro
Illustrated by Pat Cupples

A bee buzzes, a dog barks, leaves rustle in the wind. Sounds are all around us. Have you ever wondered how these sounds are made? They're caused by vibrations. Gently touch the front of your throat and say something out loud. Do you feel your vocal cords moving? Your vibrating vocal cords produce sound waves that travel through the air and into your ears.

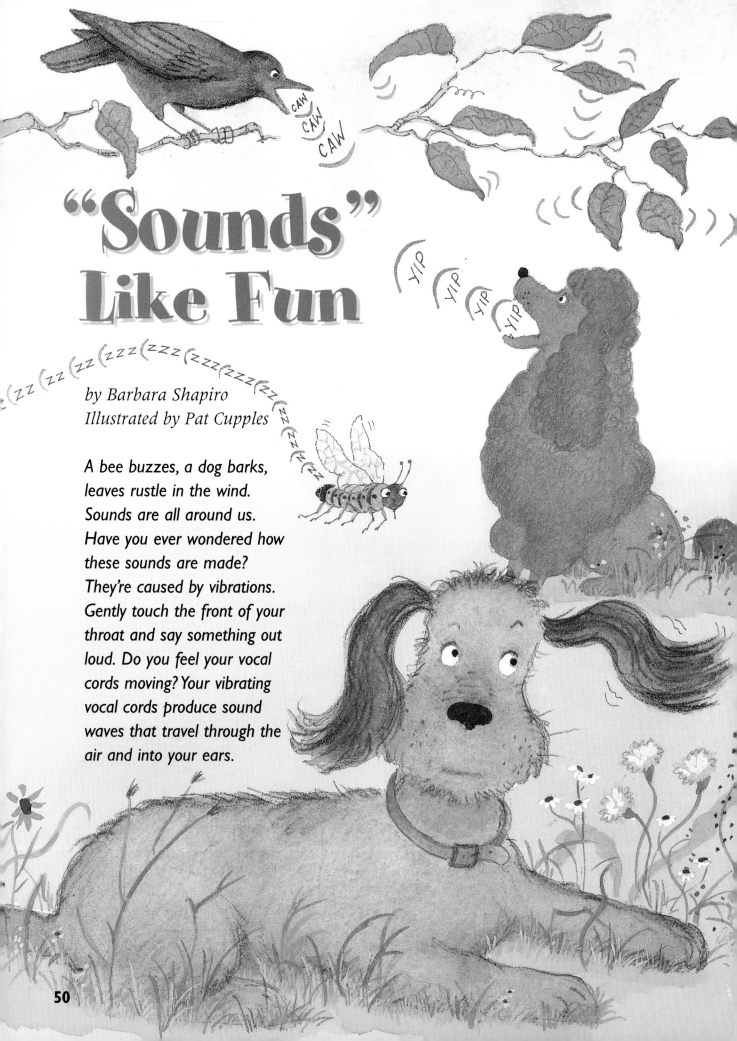

What are sound waves?

When you walk or run, the air around you moves. You push the air in front of you, and behind you air moves in to fill the space your body just left. The same thing happens when your vocal cords vibrate. They act just like a rubber band stretched between your fingers. When you pluck the centre of the rubber band, it moves back and forth, pushing the air around it. The air is made up of tiny particles called *molecules*. As the molecules of air that are next to the rubber band move, they push other molecules of air. You can see the rubber band moving, but you don't notice the air moving because it is invisible.

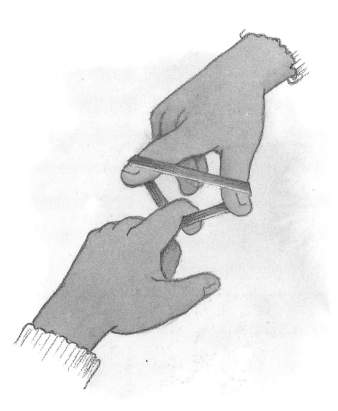

To see how air moves near a vibrating object, put about 3 cm of water into a large bowl or pan. Then drop a penny in the centre. Do you see waves of water moving away in all directions? These waves are similar to waves made in the air whenever something moves. Each wave pushes the air molecules that are near it, and another wave is formed. Sound is carried on waves of vibrating molecules. These waves are called "sound waves."

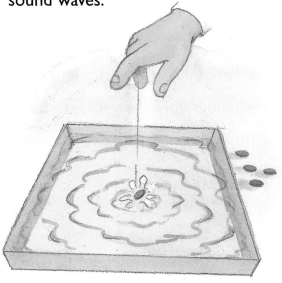

The waves of water around the penny start out strong. They get weaker as they move away. The same thing happens to sound waves as they move farther away from a plucked rubber band or another moving object. This is why a sound is louder when you are closer to where it comes from. It's also why it can't be heard at all when you are too far away.

How do we hear sound waves?

Sound waves move through the air. As they enter our ears, they push on the eardrums, sending signals to the brain where the movement is translated into sound. To see how this works, you'll need a cardboard tube from paper towels or toilet tissue, a balloon, a rubber band, and a pencil. Ask an adult for a candle and a match. Cut a piece of rubber from the balloon and stretch it across one end of the cardboard tube. Attach it with the rubber band. Then place the other end of the tube (the end without the balloon) about 3 cm away from the candle wick. You may need to rest the tube on a book to get it to the right height.

Light the candle. Then turn off the lights and tap the stretched balloon sharply with the eraser end of the pencil. Does the candle flame move?

When the balloon is tapped, it moves back and forth very quickly. This movement makes air waves inside the tube, which begin at the balloon and move through the tube and past the candle flame. These moving waves of air cause the flame to flicker.

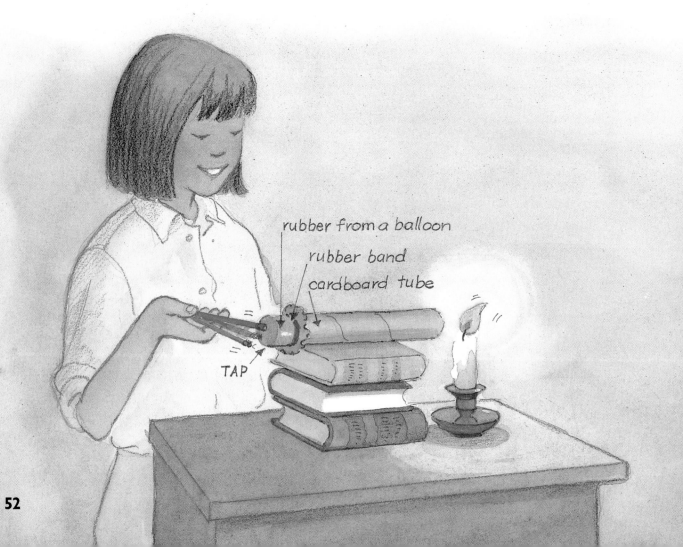

rubber from a balloon
rubber band
cardboard tube

TAP

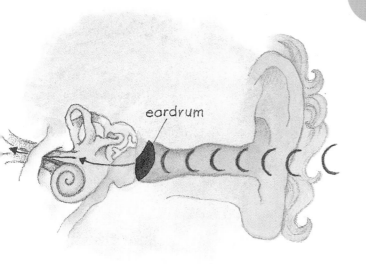

eardrum

How do we hear different sounds?

When moving waves of air enter our ears, we hear a sound. The sound's pitch depends on how fast the molecules of air are moving. Fast-moving sound waves make a high-pitched noise, like a whistle or a mosquito's buzz. Slower-moving waves make lower-pitched sounds, like the beat of a big drum.

Sometimes air molecules move too slowly or too quickly, and we can't hear them at all. The air waves made by the flap of a butterfly's wings are too slow to be heard by human ears. Some sounds, such as the cries of bats, move the air waves very quickly, making them too high-pitched for us to hear. Bats can hear them, though. Other animals, such as dogs, are also able to hear higher-pitched sounds than we can. That is one reason many hunters use dogs to help them find their prey.

Since the human eardrum is much more sensitive than a rubber balloon, moving air molecules are enough to make it vibrate. Rather than sending the sound waves through an empty cardboard tube, the ear sends them through a series of bones, tissues, and liquids. And instead of sending them to a candle flame, our ears send messages from the sound waves to our brains.

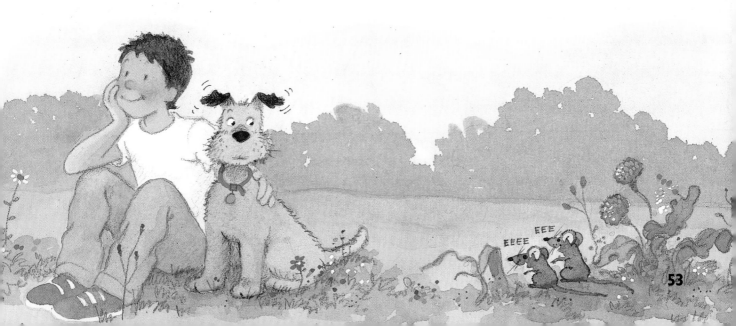

What have you learned about sound?

Think again about that bee. How does it make its buzz? What part of the bee is moving? Think about the dog. Why do some dogs have high-pitched barks and others low-pitched barks? Do their vocal cords move at different speeds? And what about those rustling leaves? Why can you only hear them if you're close by? Does it have anything to do with the distance the sound waves are able to travel through the air?

Listen carefully to the world around you, and you'll discover the answers.

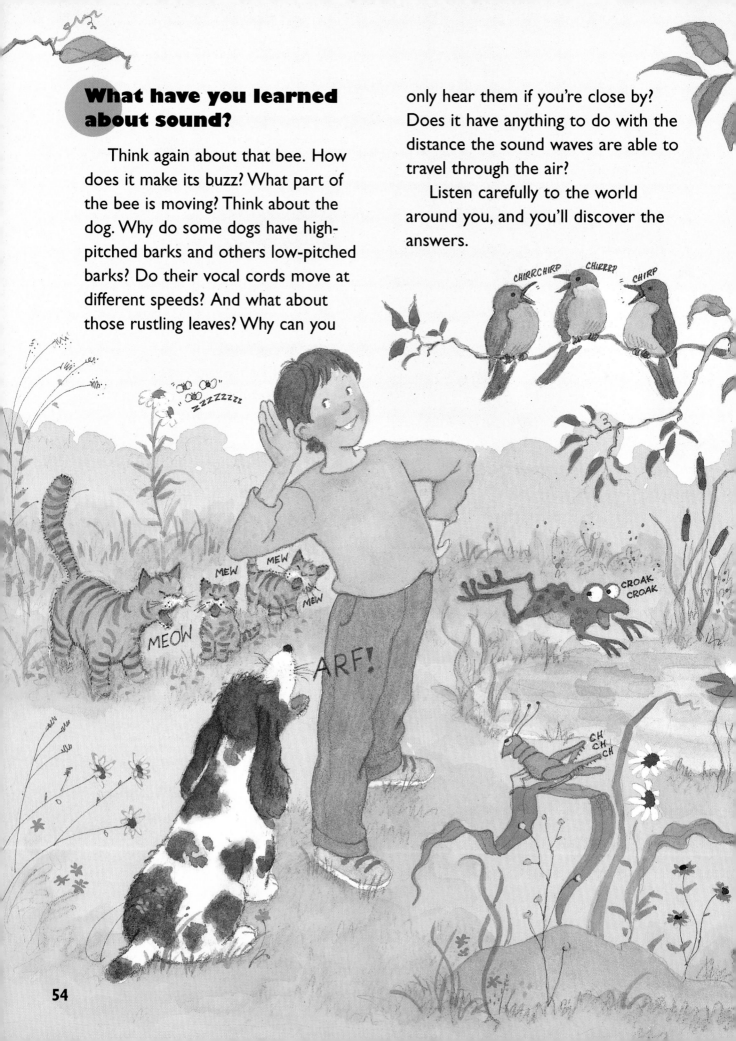

The Sweet Song

I heard a bird sing a sweet song,
Another joins and sings along.
Soon there are three,
All singing a sweet melody.
This lovely song rings in my head,
Even when I am in bed.

Pauline Voon
Age 9

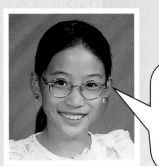

I like writing stories and poems so people can read them. Writing is fun because you can write about whatever you want and make the characters in the story do funny things.

Pauline Voon

Sounds Everywhere

I can hear sounds everywhere! I can hear sounds in my house, in school, in the grocery store, and more and more, I can hear the birds chirp in the morning. I can hear the bell buzz at school. I can hear children shout in the park. I can hear bags shuffle at the grocery store. In the house, there is the sound of my mother sweeping the floor and more and more. Sounds are everywhere!

Carmen Fong
Age 9

It is always fun writing, and I have many ideas when I write. I love writing!

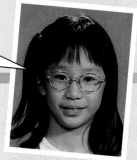

Carmen Fong

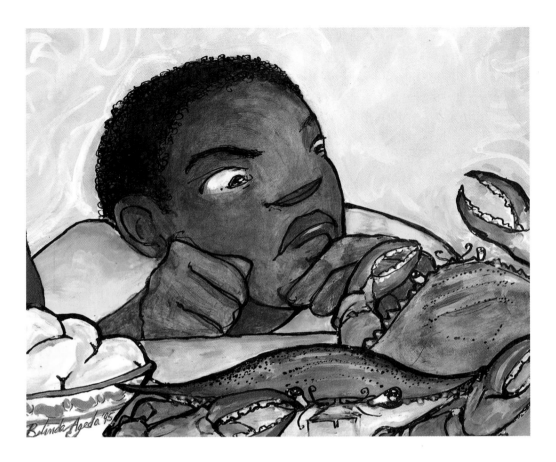

Crabs for Dinner

by Adwoa Badoe
Illustrated by Belinda Ageda

I do not like crab.
I do not like fufu.
I do not like palm nut soup.
My sister Emily does not like crab.
She does not like fufu.
She does not like palm nut soup.

So when my aunties and uncle come to dinner we eat chicken or French fries or pizza or hamburgers and we never touch the stuff the grown-ups are eating.

They eat crabs. Big grey crabs with orange-tipped pincers that Mom buys from the African shop. She makes soup with palm nut and crabs. The grown-ups eat the soup along with soft balls of potato fufu.

"Mmm," Aunt Pauline said to my mom. "No one makes crab and fufu quite like you do."

"Delicious, simply delicious," Uncle Robert said between mouthfuls of potato fufu.

My Aunt Araba's sucking and crunching sound said it all for her.

"Disgusting," Emily whispered behind Mommy's back.

"Yuk," I whispered.

One summer, my grandmother came for a visit all the way from Africa.

"Ghana," she said. "That's where I come from."

She brought us funny-looking clothes, the kind they wear in Ghana. I had a smock made of a rough cotton fabric with stripes of bright colors woven into it.

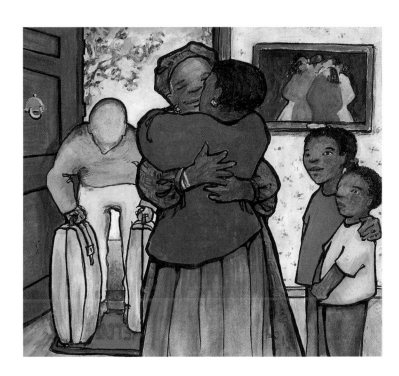

It was long and loose, almost like a dress. Grandma said it was meant to be worn over a pair of trousers.

"I'm never going to wear those," I said to my mom.

But Emily wore hers, a colorful batik dress with embroidery around the neck.

She looked so pretty that I decided to wear my smock. When I did, I thought I looked "cool." Especially when I wore the striped cotton cap that came with the smock.

Grandma had lots of stories to tell. Stories her grandmother told her when she was young. I liked the ones about a cunning "Spider man" who got in and out of all kinds of trouble.

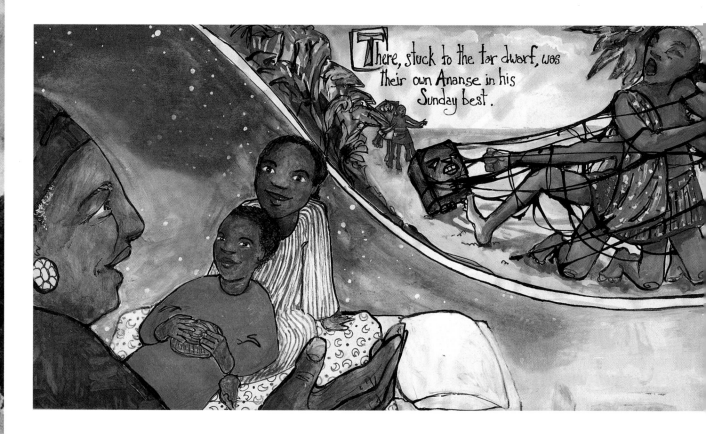

There, stuck to the tar dwarf, was their own Ananse in his Sunday best.

She always ended in a funny way, saying: "This story of mine whether good or bad, may pass away, or come to stay. It is your turn to tell your story."

So we took our turn and told her stories. And she liked them just as much as we liked hers.

A week before she left for Ghana, she invited my aunts and uncle to dinner.

"She's going to make soup and yucky crab," Emily said. "I'll bet she makes a lot of it. But I won't even take a bite."

She did make the soup, only she put in okra too.

"That's going to make it slimy," I said.

"Double Yuk," said Emily.

But dinner got cooked and dinner was served and grace was said.

Emily and I were eating hot dogs and the grown-ups were eating slime.

Uncle Robert rolled his eyes upward. "Mmm," he said. "Exquisite!"

I had never heard him use that word for Mom's soup.

"My word," Aunt Pauline said, "I had almost forgotten the original taste."

My mom simply said, "Delicious."

Even Aunt Araba paused from the sucking and crunching to say one word, "Authentic!"

I noticed that Grandma's soup smelled really good, much better than Mom's soup. Suddenly I wanted to taste just a little bit of the fufu with crab and soup.

"Can I have a little, please?" I heard Emily ask.

"Why, of course!" Grandma replied.

If Emily doesn't die, I'll have some, I thought.

Emily took a bite and didn't die. Instead she took another bite.

"And how about you?" said Grandma.

"Yes, please," I said.

It tasted different, not like the soups I knew. It was spicy and hot and really good. It was thick and smooth and I thought I could taste the flavor of ginger.

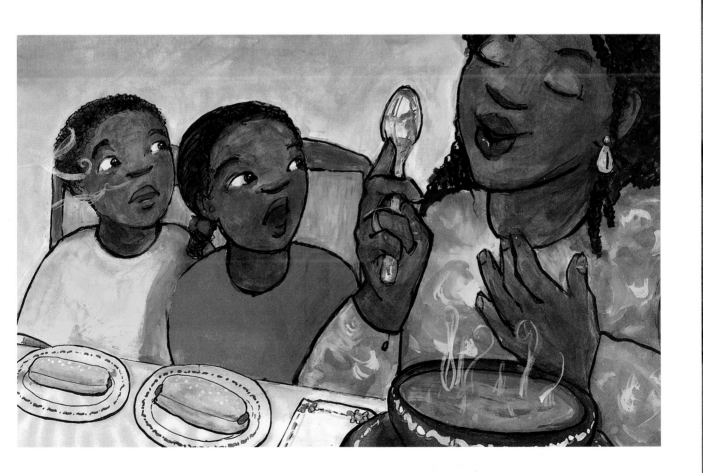

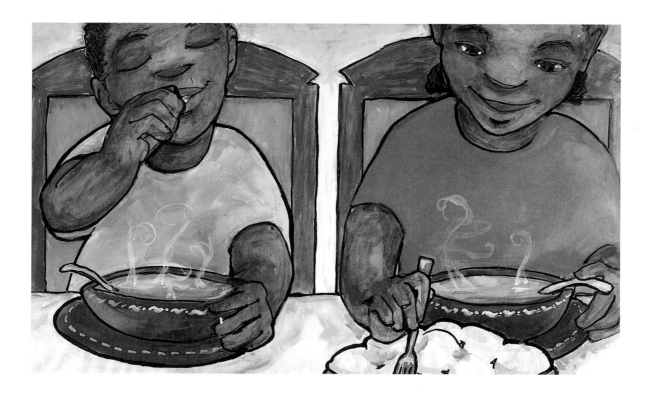

I broke off a tiny piece of crab and sucked it just like Mommy did. It was all soft inside. Then I crunched on it, really hard, just as my Aunt Araba did.

Then I ate a whole bowl of fufu and soup and a huge piece of crab.

When I was done I rolled my eyes up to the sky and said aloud, "Exquisite!"

I am not even sure what that means, but probably it is a way of saying that sometimes grandmothers cook better than mothers.

ABOUT THE ILLUSTRATOR BELINDA AGEDA

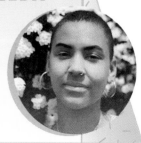

Belinda Ageda is a talented artist who is enjoying a very successful career as a book illustrator. She has also worked doing scenic paintings for theatre productions.

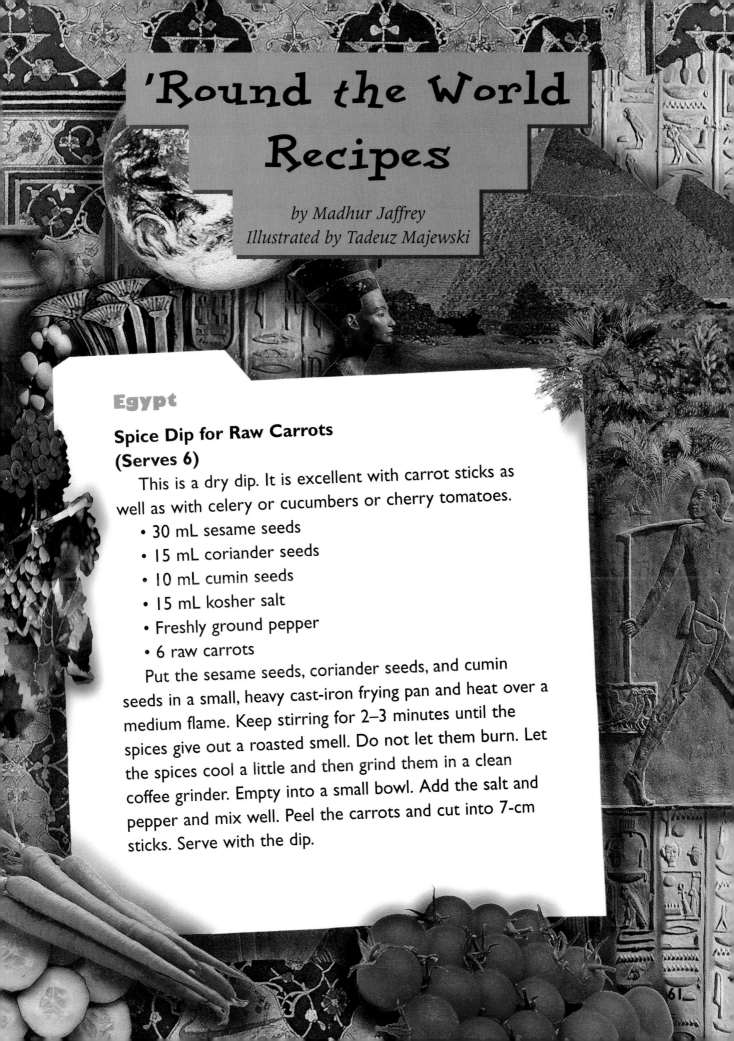

'Round the World Recipes

by Madhur Jaffrey
Illustrated by Tadeuz Majewski

Egypt

Spice Dip for Raw Carrots
(Serves 6)

This is a dry dip. It is excellent with carrot sticks as well as with celery or cucumbers or cherry tomatoes.

- 30 mL sesame seeds
- 15 mL coriander seeds
- 10 mL cumin seeds
- 15 mL kosher salt
- Freshly ground pepper
- 6 raw carrots

Put the sesame seeds, coriander seeds, and cumin seeds in a small, heavy cast-iron frying pan and heat over a medium flame. Keep stirring for 2–3 minutes until the spices give out a roasted smell. Do not let them burn. Let the spices cool a little and then grind them in a clean coffee grinder. Empty into a small bowl. Add the salt and pepper and mix well. Peel the carrots and cut into 7-cm sticks. Serve with the dip.

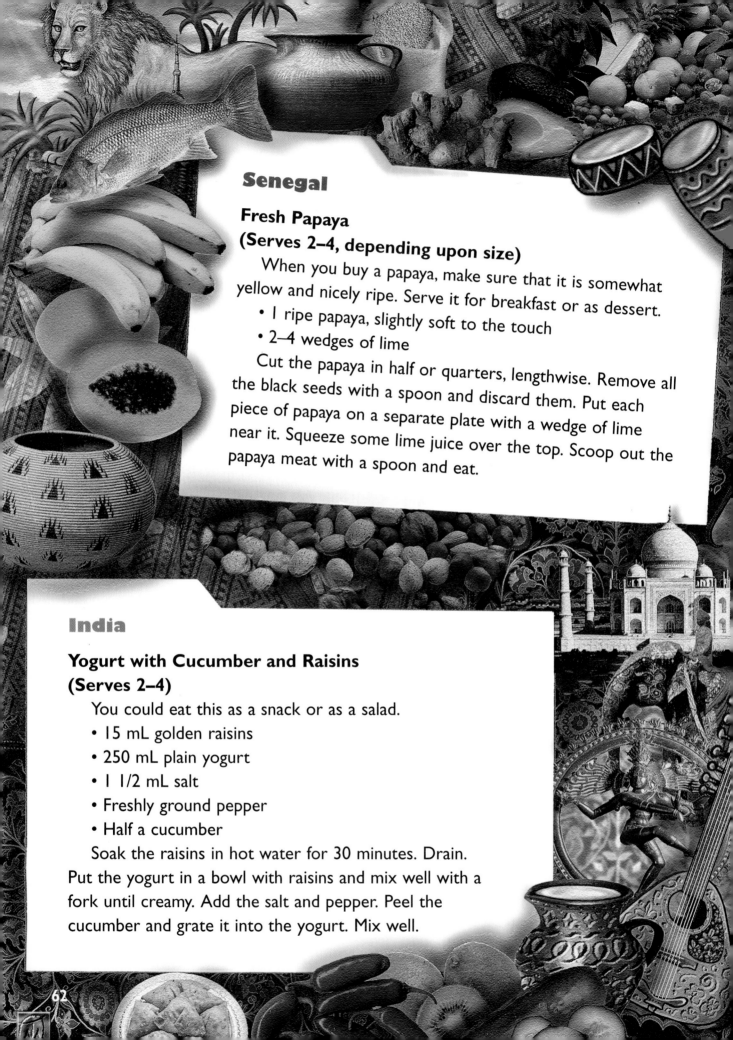

Senegal

Fresh Papaya
(Serves 2–4, depending upon size)

When you buy a papaya, make sure that it is somewhat yellow and nicely ripe. Serve it for breakfast or as dessert.

- 1 ripe papaya, slightly soft to the touch
- 2–4 wedges of lime

Cut the papaya in half or quarters, lengthwise. Remove all the black seeds with a spoon and discard them. Put each piece of papaya on a separate plate with a wedge of lime near it. Squeeze some lime juice over the top. Scoop out the papaya meat with a spoon and eat.

India

Yogurt with Cucumber and Raisins
(Serves 2–4)

You could eat this as a snack or as a salad.

- 15 mL golden raisins
- 250 mL plain yogurt
- 1 1/2 mL salt
- Freshly ground pepper
- Half a cucumber

Soak the raisins in hot water for 30 minutes. Drain. Put the yogurt in a bowl with raisins and mix well with a fork until creamy. Add the salt and pepper. Peel the cucumber and grate it into the yogurt. Mix well.

Italy

Bruschetta
(Serves 4)

You may serve this as a first course or as a snack.

- 8 slices of fresh, crusty French or Italian white bread
- About 45–60 mL olive oil
- 16 fresh basil leaves
- 250 mL chopped fresh, ripe tomatoes
- Salt
- Freshly ground pepper

Just before eating, spread the bread slices in front of you on the counter. Brush each with a little olive oil. Put two basil leaves on top of the oil. Put about 30 mL of the chopped tomatoes on top of the basil leaves. Sprinkle a little salt and pepper over the top of the tomatoes and serve.

Mexico

Tacos
(Serves 2–4)

Here is a complete meal. All that is needed afterward is some fruit.

- 175 mL canned black beans
- 4 taco shells
- 60 mL shredded cheese (Cheddar or Monterey Jack) – optional
- 60 mL shredded lettuce
- 60 mL chopped tomatoes
- Salt
- Freshly ground pepper

Put the beans in a bowl and mash them lightly. Put 45 mL of the mashed beans in each taco shell. Put 15 mL of shredded cheese (optional) on top of the beans in each shell. Top the cheese with 15 mL each of the lettuce and then the tomatoes. Sprinkle a little salt and pepper on the tomatoes and serve immediately.

Touch It, Taste It

by Gordon Penrose
Photographed by Ray Boudreau

What Happens?

There are nerves under your skin that send messages to your brain. They help you feel different things. When you squeeze the nails, your nerves feel both the hot and cold, but they have a hard time telling them apart because the two different temperatures are so close together. So, your nerves send your brain a "tingling" feeling instead.

Temperature Trick

1. Put a nail in a cup of hot tap water. Put another nail in cold water.
2. After a few minutes, take them out. Then squeeze the nails in your hand. What do you feel?

Add salt to a grapefruit and make it taste...sweeter?

1. Separate a grapefruit into pieces, and sprinkle a bit of salt on one piece.
2. Taste an unsalted piece. Then try a salted piece. What a difference!

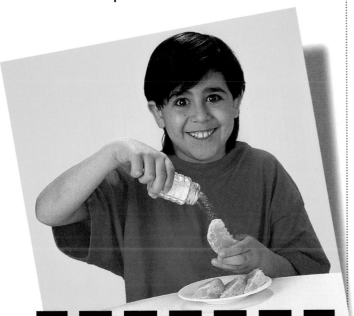

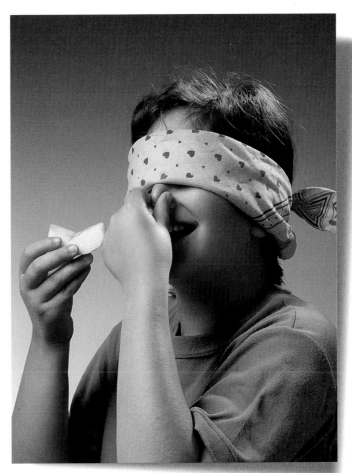

What Happens?

Your tongue only tastes sweet, sour, salty, and bitter flavors. Grapefruit tastes sour and salt tastes salty, but when you taste them together the salt flavor stops you from tasting as much of the sour flavor. So, the salted grapefruit seems less sour than the unsalted one.

Taste Test

Which would you rather eat, a raw potato or a raw apple? Take a taste test to find out. Here's how:

1. Start with peeled slices of uncooked potato and apple.
2. Cover your eyes with a blindfold.
3. Tightly hold your nose with one hand.
4. Take a bite of each slice. Can you tell which is which?

Try the same test with fruit juice.

Hold your nose and take a sip of grape juice, then of apple juice. Can you tell them apart?

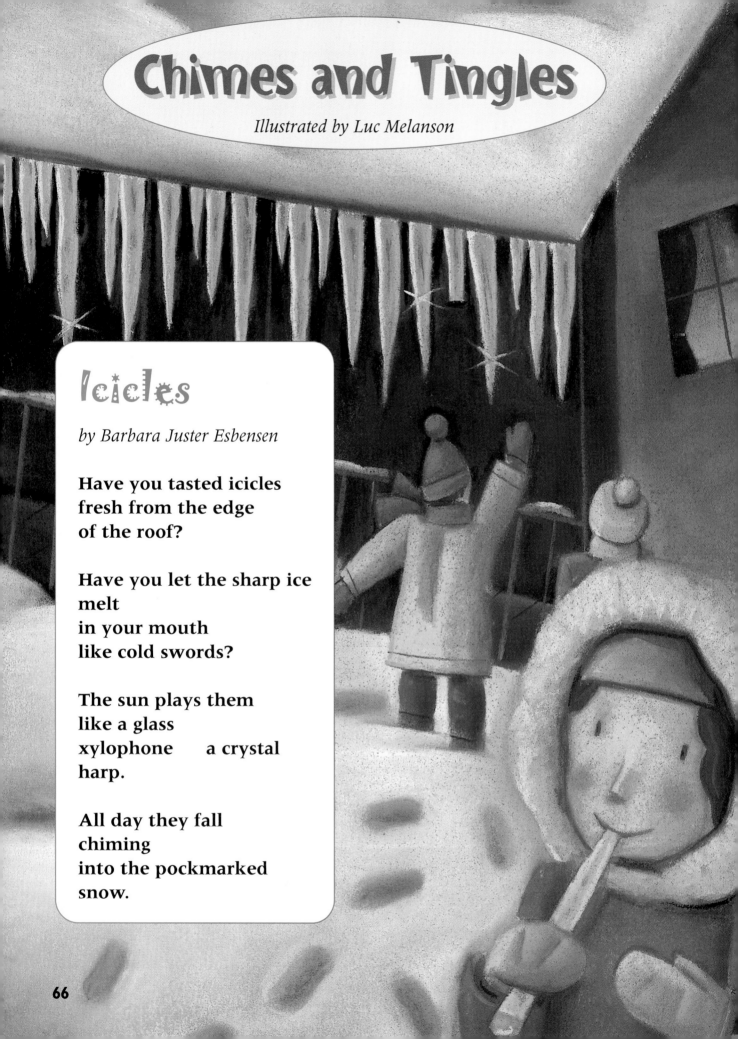

Chimes and Tingles

Illustrated by Luc Melanson

Icicles

by Barbara Juster Esbensen

Have you tasted icicles
fresh from the edge
of the roof?

Have you let the sharp ice
melt
in your mouth
like cold swords?

The sun plays them
like a glass
xylophone   a crystal
harp.

All day they fall
chiming
into the pockmarked
snow.

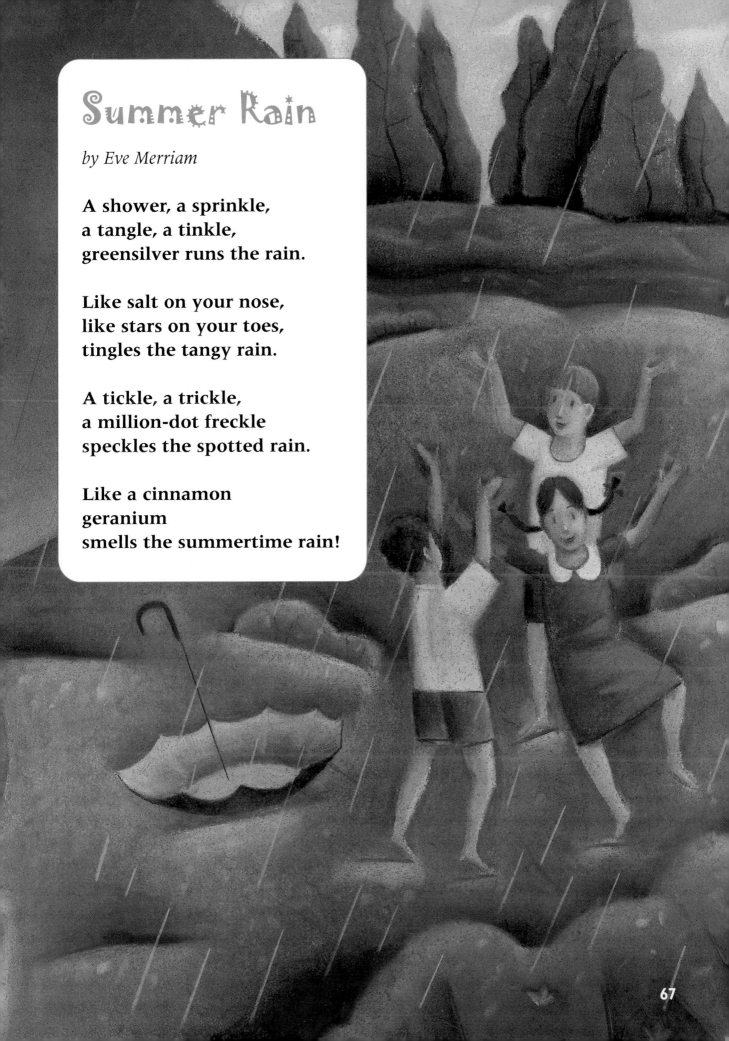

Summer Rain

by Eve Merriam

A shower, a sprinkle,
a tangle, a tinkle,
greensilver runs the rain.

Like salt on your nose,
like stars on your toes,
tingles the tangy rain.

A tickle, a trickle,
a million-dot freckle
speckles the spotted rain.

Like a cinnamon
geranium
smells the summertime rain!

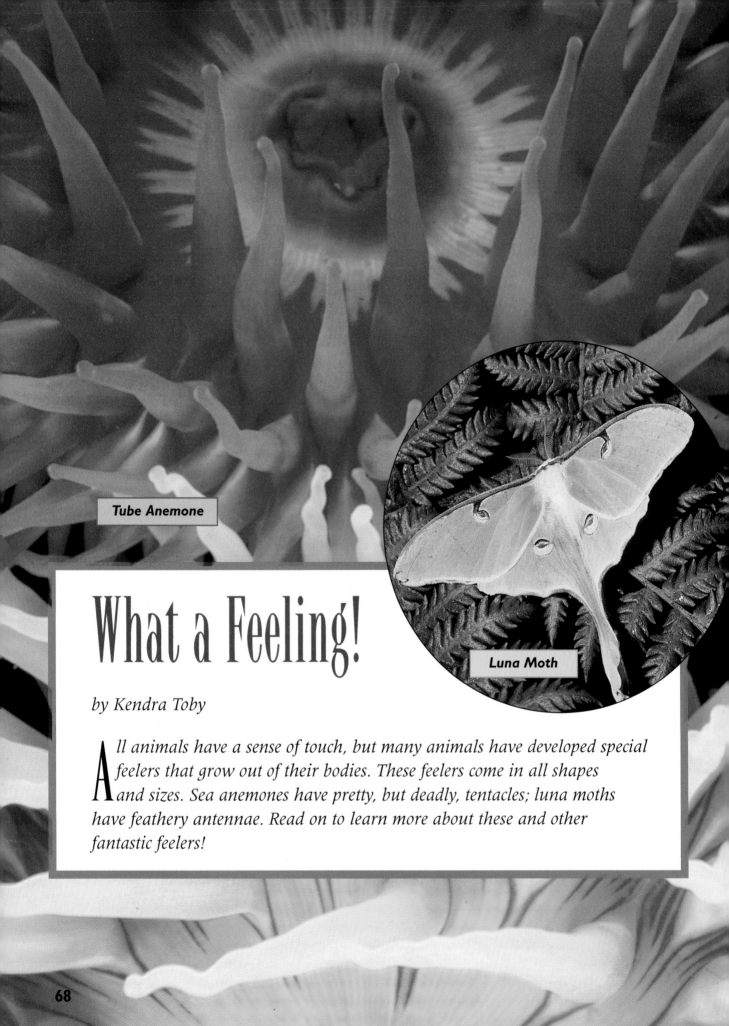

Tube Anemone

Luna Moth

What a Feeling!

by Kendra Toby

All animals have a sense of touch, but many animals have developed special feelers that grow out of their bodies. These feelers come in all shapes and sizes. Sea anemones have pretty, but deadly, tentacles; luna moths have feathery antennae. Read on to learn more about these and other fantastic feelers!

Touchy Tentacles

What's this huge, hairy mess floating in the open ocean? Is it a creature from outer space? No, it's a lion's mane, the world's largest jellyfish. Its slithery, slimy body can be as big as a trampoline. But even at that size, there's not much to it—just a mouth and a stomach. Lion's mane jellyfish have more than 150 tentacles to "see" and capture prey.

The tentacles usually do nothing but hang in the water, waiting for supper. Each one can be as long as a telephone pole. When an unlucky fish, shrimp, or crab touches a tentacle—ZAP!

Small capsules called nematocysts (nee-MAH-tuh-sists) located all over the jellyfish's tentacles shoot out tiny darts, called barbs, that hook into the prey. The barbs contain powerful poison that paralyzes the unlucky target. Then the lion's mane slowly pulls the prey into its mouth with its long tentacles.

All jellyfish have tentacles and barbs, but none are as poisonous as the lion's mane. Sea anemones also use tentacles and barbs to feel around and capture food.

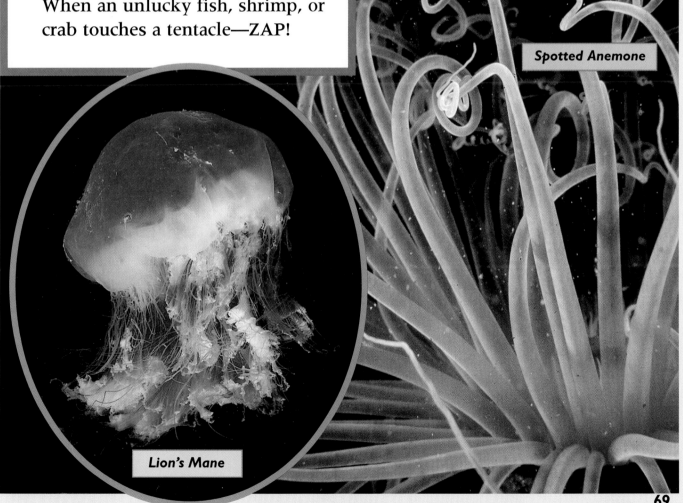

Spotted Anemone

Lion's Mane

The Blue Browsers

Fish that lurk on the dark bottoms of rivers and oceans need more than eyes to find food. For this job, blue catfish have special feelers called barbels (BAR-bels). Four pairs of barbels stick out from the fish's nose, jaw, and chin. While the eyes of this scary-looking creature are watching out for enemies, its barbels sweep the river bottom, feeling for a tasty meal of fish.

Catfish aren't the only fish that use barbels to feel their way around. Ocean species, such as the hairy blenny and Atlantic cod, also have barbels. Blue goatfish have two long, ribbonlike barbels hanging down from below their jaw. When they're not using them to find food, they tuck them away back under their chin.

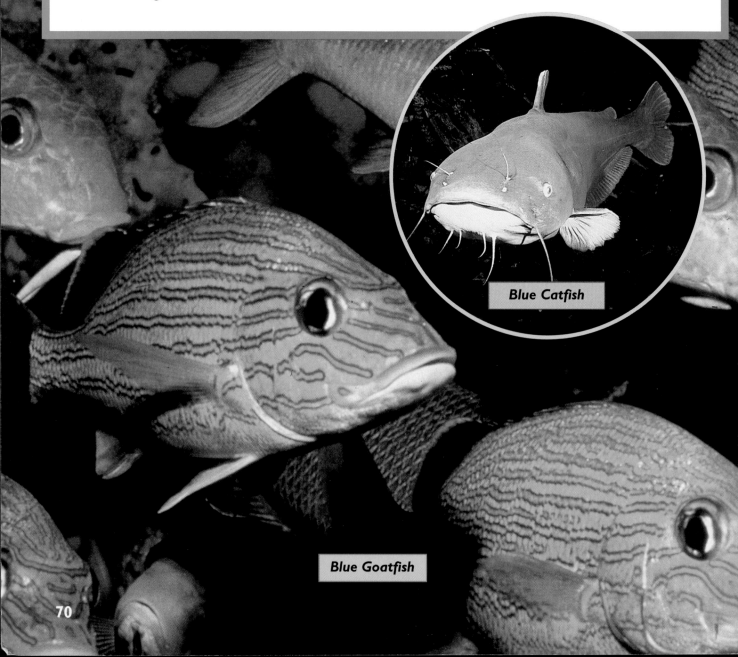

Blue Catfish

Blue Goatfish

Bird Bristles

Some birds have bristles for feeling and trapping insects at night. The owlet nightjar is a nocturnal species that lives in Australia. The elaborate feelers around its beak are actually special feathers called semi-bristles. They help the bird find and scoop up insects as it flies through the air.

You don't have to go as far as Australia to find birds with bristles. The whip-poor-will is a type of nightjar that lives in southern Canada. It uses its bristles to feel and trap insects.

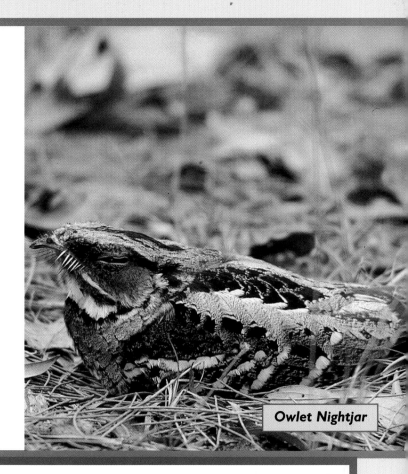

Owlet Nightjar

Winning Whiskers

Did you know that all mammals except humans use whiskers to feel with?

Walruses and seals are animals that use their whiskers to feel along the ocean bottom for crabs, mollusks, sea urchins, squid, and fish.

When whiskers touch an object, thousands of nerve fibers under the skin tell the brain what the object feels like, how big it is, and what shape it is.

As you can see, being in touch with the environment is important for all living things. Now you have a "feel" for some of nature's fantastic feelers!

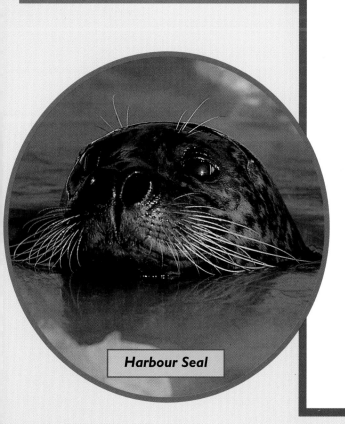

Harbour Seal

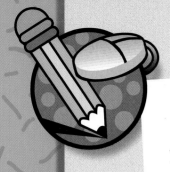

Touch

It was my fourth birthday.
The shiny sparklers on my cake tempted me.
My mom said, "Don't touch!"
My dad said, "Don't touch!"
My friends said, "Don't touch!"
I touched, "Ouch!!!"

Kyle Fontaine
Age 9

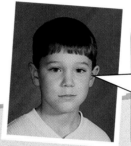

Kyle Fontaine

When my teacher asked me to write a poem about touch, I remembered the pain of hot sparklers on my fourth birthday. My finger was burnt so badly that I could not open my presents. Luckily, my friend Tim helped me open my presents.

The Skunk

Once there was a boy named Marc. When he was little there was a skunk on the loose near his house. His mom said, "If you see an animal that looks like a black and white cat don't smell it." His dad said the same thing. But Marc didn't listen. When he saw the skunk he went right up to it. Pwww! The skunk sprayed him with a stinky smell. Time for a bath in tomato juice!

Ross Cook
Age 9

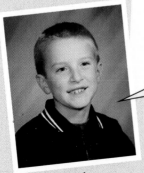

Ross Cook

I think that it is a big honor having my story read by so many people.